Lift Yourself

Born and raised in Surrey, Laura Hoggins developed her passion for lifting after discovering a CrossFit box in Hammersmith over three years ago. Inspired by the community of individuals whose priority was athletics and not their aesthetic, Laura quit her office job and moved into fitness full time. Now a fully trained fitness coach and personal trainer, Laura runs her own concept class, LIFTED, at the Ministry of Sound Fitness. Laura has over 18,000 Instagram followers and has worked with British Women's Lifting, Women in Sport and This Girl Can to spread a campaign that she supports that 'strong is not a size'. Runner-up in the Men's Health Gym Awards '18 for Smartest Coach, and a regular contributor to *Women's Health, Metro* and *Health & Fitness Magazine*, Laura speaks on podcasts, at festivals and events across the country and is the female face celebrating lifting in the UK. She recently launched her own podcast, Biceps and Banter.

@laurabiceps
https://www.lifted.fitness/

Lift Yourself

A Training Guide to Getting Fit and
Feeling Strong for Life

LAURA HOGGINS

PENGUIN LIFE

AN IMPRINT OF

PENGUIN BOOKS

PENGUIN LIFE

UK | USA | Canada | Ireland | Australia
India | New Zealand | South Africa

Penguin Life is part of the Penguin Random House group of companies
whose addresses can be found at global.penguinrandomhouse.com.

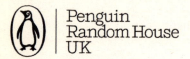

First published 2019
001

Set in 12/14.75pt Dante MT Std
Typeset by Jouve (UK), Milton Keynes
Printed and bound in Great Britain by Clays Ltd, Elcograf S.p.A.

A CIP catalogue record for this book is available from the British Library

ISBN: 978–0–241–38591–3

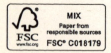

Contents

To anyone who has ever felt
they were not good enough,
not thin enough,
not fast enough,
not strong enough,
not confident enough.

You are more than enough.
Only you decide.
Take control.

1. LIFT-OFF

Lifting changed my life, and I believe it has the power to change yours too.

So, what do I mean by lifting? At its simplest, it's just that: building strength by lifting things. Essentially, you're using resistance to stimulate muscle contractions to make you stronger. The resistance you use can be weights that you hold, weight machines at the gym, resistance bands or even your own body weight (think of the resistance you're using when you do a press-up or a plank, for example). There are many different ways in which you can use your body weight or do resistance training to build strength; the fun part is figuring out which way you want to do it.

There's zero doubt that we should all be building our own versions of strength training into our weekly schedules. Decades of research have shown us that it can reduce your body fat, improve your posture, protect your bones and heart, make you happier and help you live longer. That's quite a list. The NHS now advises everyone to do two sessions of strength training every week, sessions that work all the major muscle groups. That's alongside the 150 minutes of weekly aerobic (or 'cardio') activity we're all supposed to do, such as walking, running, cycling, or playing sport.

If you're now thinking – hang on, two sessions, really? – you're not alone. According to the Health Survey for England in 2016, roughly two-thirds of us are managing to hit the cardio target, but only 31 per cent of men and 23 per cent of women do any muscle-strengthening work. There are many reasons for this, and I see it every day in my work as a personal trainer, which is why I am so passionate about trying to open people up to the wonders of being strong:

- We're cardio junkies. For years, women in particular have assumed that doing endless cardio exercise – running, hanging out on the cross-trainer, bashing out a bit of the old step aerobics – is the only way they're going to keep their weight under control and increase their fitness. I once thought that too; I spent hours on the flippin' cross-trainer and used to walk past the weights area like 'whatever' . . . but I was wrong, and this book will show you why.

- Lifting seems complicated. Yes, there is a bit more to it than just lacing up your trainers and nipping outside for a run or walk, but it doesn't actually have to be difficult.

- Gyms can be intimidating. Especially the weights area, which is often full of big men who look like they know what they're doing.

I'm going to address all these potential barriers in this book and show you that lifting needn't be complicated or intimidating, and that you don't even need to go to the gym to do it.

Lifting is incredibly empowering, and it makes you both physically and mentally stronger. There's also an addictive element to it that appeals to my inner warrior, and it might speak to yours too. That feeling of lifting something you didn't think you could . . . it not only makes you look like a total boss, but I promise you'll feel like one too. I'm also going to share my personal journey with you. I hope that by being totally transparent, there will be bits you can relate to, and then maybe my experience can help you too.

Ten years ago, I was dragging myself out of bed with just about enough time to get some mascara on plus a bit of dry shampoo, and then off I'd go to the office for another day hunched over my desk, probably having a cigarette on the way. I was unhappy with my body, and over the years I'd tried every diet going – and I mean every single one.

Then I discovered lifting and my whole mindset changed. I began celebrating what my body could do rather than criticizing how it looked. Fast-forward to the present and I'm now a personal trainer working in some of London's top gyms. I was honoured to be named runner-up in the smart coach category of the 2018 Men's Health Gym Awards, and it's been my absolute privilege to work on the #StrongIsNotASize campaign, alongside GB Olympic weightlifter Zoe Smith, to encourage more women into lifting, driven by British Weight Lifting and the charity Women in Sport. I want to show you that loving your body instead of trying to sabotage yourself can give you a whole new perspective on life.

All around us the culture is changing. Over the years I have been inspired by many prominent figures. People like Joslyn Thompson Rule, Lisa Price, Anna-Maria Ronnqvist, Joe Wicks, Alice Liveing, Bradley Simmonds, Donna Moore and Chloe Madeley are showing just how accessible weights can be, alongside a community of female fans who are finding each other through hashtags like #womenwholift and #strongwoman. Anna-Maria Ronnqvist, a colleague, inspiration and close friend of mine who just happens to be Strongwoman World Champion of 2017 and 2018, can lift more than twice her body weight. Now, I'm not expecting you to be able to do the same, although I would love nothing more than to inspire a future weightlifting champion. I certainly can't lift that kind of weight and I've spent years training.

What I am NOT about to tell you is how to turn into a Victoria's Secret model, how to sculpt yourself the bottom of a Kardashian or how to get 'ripped' for Ibiza in 36 hours, all by eating kale steamed five million ways or by drinking herbal infusions. I don't really like kale and I certainly don't want to steam it, there isn't a detox tea in the world that will turn you into Kim Kardashian, and being 'beach body ready' just isn't my jam, especially not overnight, unless you fancy sleeping in a sauna (not advised!).

What I can show you is how to set realistic goals and find your rhythm so you can discover what lifting can do for you. Lifting isn't about quick fixes – although I do believe that if you train just twice a week you could see and feel change and progress in only four weeks. It's about developing a strong body and mind, and being able to set yourself on a path so you can keep training when you're sixty, just like my amazing mum (more on her later). It really is training for life.

How to use this book

You may be reading this because you are a total beginner and have never lifted anything apart from your shopping. Or maybe you once tried lifting but struggled to keep it up. Or perhaps you've done some training but didn't see results. Whether you haven't even tried to lift a weight yet or whether you're an experienced lifter looking for some guidance, this book is for you. I will cover:

- The amazing benefits of lifting
- My ten commandments for lifting . . . and life

- How to lift safely and effectively

- How to set goals and monitor your progress

- The key functional moves you need to know about

But first, I want to start by sharing with you a bit about myself, about how I got here, and why the journey I took could benefit you, too.

My personal journey

If you had told me ten years ago that I would be writing a book on how to get fit and lift weights, I would have laughed so hard I would have probably given myself some accidental rock-solid abs. The irony!

I remember a time when I was uncomfortable with what I saw in the mirror. I didn't look like the women on the covers of magazines (fitness or otherwise) and I felt overweight and discontented with myself. For years I drank a lot, partied a lot and smoked way too much. I managed to lose weight . . . but then managed to gain it all back again. I spent years on diets; I've done them all.

Going back even further, I was always a sporty child. At six I began kicking a football around the park with my cousin, and at school I begged to be allowed to train with the boys. Girls just didn't do football then, so I was always the only girl on the pitch, with my sleeves so long they hung down over my hands and my football socks up to my thighs. But I loved it: working together as a team and cheering each other on, win or lose. As a teenager I was invited to join Chelsea Under-16 girls team, which was an absolute honour. I was small, but I was pretty fast, agile and relatively powerful.

By the time I was 16 I was working part-time in a commercial gym in Weybridge, Surrey. I thought I'd work there for ever, but I got good grades at college and I guess the next expected step was university. When it came to the application deadline I still had no clue what I was going to study, so I copied the course code from my friend Jo, which happened to be business studies and marketing. Bizarrely, I got in. It's not exactly the sort of solid careers advice you'd give your children, but hey, it led me to the world of business and retail. So it was sort of by accident that I had a ten-year corporate career where I ended up being in charge of a turnover of millions.

I had never been happy with my size, even as a teenager, and I'd become 'university fat' – the result of eating badly, lack of sleep and too many pints of cider far too often. So by the time I started my first job, working in marketing for Unilever, I felt pretty unhappy in my body. I'm only 5 foot 3 inches, so I felt like I couldn't carry very much extra weight.

Over the years I must have tried every diet going, from Keto, Paleo, Atkins and 5:2 to trying to live off nuts and seeds. You name it, I tried it. Sometimes I lost weight, sometimes I put on weight. But I'd got into that place that some of you may recognize, where the scales dictate your whole life. I was obsessed with my weight every waking hour. If I only ate almonds today, would I lose a pound? If I skipped breakfast and only drank smoothies for a few days, would I be any slimmer? My whole ambition was to get to 8.5 stone. If I could only do that I would be happy. There's so much wrong with that mindset, I hardly know where to start! I'll be addressing the whole area of goals and mindsets later in the book and sharing more of my personal experiences. Just so you know, that is certainly no longer my goal – I am nowhere near 8.5 stone and I've never felt fitter, stronger or happier in my own skin than I do right now.

It wasn't just the stress and the crazy eating habits where I was getting it wrong. I was also partying hard, smoking and drinking. Every weekend I was out with friends and colleagues, drinking mindlessly and crawling into bed in the early hours. In truth I think I got comfortable being stressed out, stuck in a cycle of making bad decisions for my health and then looking for a temporary escape in partying.

Then one day I suddenly realized I wasn't enjoying myself any more. I was at my absolute heaviest, I was binge drinking, I was not eating well, and the turbulent relationship with my long-term boyfriend had ended badly. It felt like a moment when something had to give. My parents were living in the Cayman Islands at the time, so I decided to leave everything behind, make a fresh start and move there. In the year I was there, I lived a simple, active, healthy and non-materialistic lifestyle. I lost on average 1lb a week because I was so active, which meant that I lost about 50lb, or 3.5 stone, just by eating simply, not being stressed and working outside on the boats. But most important-ly, I found my fire again. I wasn't weighing myself religiously any more; I felt good, so I didn't care.

Invigorated, I moved back to London and back to my cor-porate job. I was back to being sedentary at a desk job but I had a new sense of purpose, so at the same time, I threw myself into fitness. However, I did the only thing I knew how to do: basically running, running and more running. Like most of us, I'd grown up thinking cardio exercise was the only way to get fit and lose weight, and I was still two stone off that 'ideal' weight I'd set myself. Being back home in London, I started to care about that goal of being 8.5 stone again.

I changed jobs and went to work at L'Oreal, where I enjoyed an amazing five-year career. It was a huge learning curve for me, and somehow I ended up the lead account manager for Maybelline Cosmetics. Again, I wasn't quite sure if this was my path – and even less so when the director interviewing me asked me to empty out my make-up bag and talk her through the contents, and what colour I used on my hair. I only had a few bits and a basic mascara – I was a sporty girl not known for my cosmetic creativity. What probably saved me was my encyclopedic knowledge of hair products and fake tan. (It may shock you to learn that I am not actually a natural blonde, or a natural orange.)

In so many ways my job at L'Oreal was incredible: I worked with some exceptional people and got to work on one of the most dynamic brands in the market. I was responsible for managing the profit-and-loss figures for thousands of products and planning exciting future product launches. But I have to admit the workload was relentless and the pressure was immense. I was either constantly travelling or sitting for long hours at my desk in head office, hunched over a screen, hitting myself over the head with PowerPoint presentations and drowning in Excel spreadsheets. My posture was diabolical, I had no core muscles and my nutritional habits were bizarre, to say the least.

It's quite an experience working in such a glamorous office. Everyone always looked amazing, and we were constantly experimenting with the latest lip colours, hair spray or (my favourite!) gradual tan. But we were also continually on some kind of diet (mainly coffee and cigarettes, in truth). There was one time a colleague and I decided we would eat one almond – yes, just the one – every half hour. And nothing else. It's so bad it seems funny now.

In 2013, four years after returning from the Cayman Islands, I entered the London Marathon. I will be totally honest with you; it wasn't for my passion of pavement pounding or to raise money, it was because I thought it would make me thinner. I reckoned that if I told my friends, family and colleagues that I was doing it, it would force me to train and I'd definitely lose weight. In two years I ran two full marathons and eight half marathons, just to get to a certain weight that seems utterly random (and unimportant) now.

Finally, I made it. The scales told me I was 8.5 stone. So was I happy to be 120lb at last? Yes, for about 20 minutes. Then I remembered I still wasn't eating properly and I was as weak as hell. I still had no core muscles, stick arms and not much definition at all to my body. I was a kind of weird 'skinny fat', if you know what I mean.

My life changed for ever when a new gym opened right opposite the office. A friend told me he was really getting into this thing called CrossFit and thought I would like it. So I went along. CrossFit, for those of you who haven't had the pleasure, is a pretty intense group training session that uses weights, barbells, kettlebells, dumbbells, ropes and all sorts of other gym equipment for an hour's workout. What's in that workout changes every day and is programmed specifically for the members of that 'Box'. Everyone in the class does the same workout, scaled to their ability. Then afterwards, while you're quietly dying on the floor, you have to shout out the time you managed to do it in and which weights you used. Your score is written up on the board for all to see for the rest of the day. Sounds brutal, right?

I turned up, absolutely terrified by what was about to happen. Sara, the beautiful and athletic coach, demonstrated each movement with pace and ease, and told me it would be just fine – if I didn't stop. Just keep going, she said. So I did. And yes, I felt like I was going to die. That was probably one of the hardest workouts I have ever done, but I wanted to finish it so badly. There was something about it: that feeling of achieve-ment to pick something up, lift it and push it above your head. It felt like success. I felt a sense of exhilaration and raw physical achievement. I couldn't wait to go back for more. No one cared what you looked like or what size you were, they just cared about your attitude. I could hardly move for days after that first class, but it was the kind of pain that felt like I'd actually done something positive with my body, even though I was scarred mentally from attempting a box jump. What an achievement! I had never considered my body to have 'achieved' anything before. I am extremely grateful for that day. I took a step into the unknown and I came out absolutely buzzing. Lifting was going to be my thing, I was sure of it.

Straight away, I enrolled in a month-long CrossFit founda-tions course and nailed the basic movement patterns and lifts, and have never looked back. I just wanted to get better at it and for the first time in my life I had a new goal that didn't revolve around my waistline or a number on the scales.

I was still working as hard as ever at L'Oreal, but now I was getting into the CrossFit Box every day at 6am for an hour's workout before heading into the office for 8am, Black-berry in hand, checking emails as I walked. I started to feel better at work, I slept better, I dealt with stress and anxiety better. I even began to eat better as I realized that a handful of almonds wasn't going to fuel my body for the serious workout it was undergoing.

In CrossFit I also found an incredible community of sup-portive and like-minded people. Most of them had a story to tell about why they were there. Maybe they'd had a moment when they suddenly realized they weren't happy in their lives, that they were prioritizing the wrong things or they lacked a certain direction or focus. But in each other we found a rock-solid support network, willing one another on to do that little bit better each day.

For me, one of the biggest eye-openers of lifting weights at CrossFit was that I regularly failed, a lot. They're designed to be tough workouts, and I often couldn't complete everything. That's the point: it's not a quick fix. You fail, then you fail again but you keep going, knowing that one day you will achieve. And when that moment comes I can't tell you how sweet it is. It was a big lesson for me, understanding that I could fail one day but it didn't mean it was all over, or that I was a failure as a person. If only I'd managed to have that attitude with all the diets I'd tried over the years!

Slowly, I began to gravitate away from my old lifestyle. I soon realized that if I wanted to be good at CrossFit, maybe it wasn't the best idea to get hammered the night before, turning up the next morning to just drag myself through the session. So I didn't go out as much any more, and as with any lifestyle change it took a bit of time for my friends to get used to it. I stopped smoking, too, as it just made me slower.

My new-found sense of contentment led me to take on a new job working for Thea Green, founder of Nails Inc, the New York-style nail bars. She's an exceptional woman, a mother and true entrepreneur who would work day and night to chase opportunities to build her business globally. It was an incredible can-do atmosphere. What I learned from her was that anything was possible. If you had a dream, you had to go for it. Hard work and perseverance would get you there.

For the first time I could see that I might be able to run my own business. I'd got my qualifications as a personal trainer and I had been taking on a few clients in the early mornings before work and at the weekends. But my big dream was to spread the message about lifting, to introduce weights to complete beginners in a supportive group atmosphere. I wanted people to feel what I'd felt about lifting that very first time: the sense of power and accomplishment. I came up with the concept of a class called LIFTED: men and women lifting weights together to big tunes, safely, just having fun. I asked the CrossFit guys if I could use the gym for two hours on a Sunday afternoon and posted on Instagram (to my eleven or so followers) that I was launching this session and that if anyone wanted to come, just let me know. I felt I was bridging a gap between gym fitness and the hardcore CrossFit that people had heard about. I got so many positive messages and was genuinely just so excited that people wanted to come and train with me and share my passion.

Six people came that first Sunday. I was so happy. I wrote 'LIFTED' on the blackboard and drafted a little session plan and we were off. A few of them posted videos on Instagram, people got super-engaged and word soon spread. It was like a secret but accessible society – soon it became so popular that I had to run two Sunday classes; I loved it.

Finally, I worked up the courage to quit my job and pursue the dream I'd had since I was fifteen, to work full-time in fitness. I got there in the end, with a slight (well, ten-year) detour. People thought I was mad to risk everything I had worked for over so many years, but the truth is I've never looked back – I can't even imagine working at a desk now. I now run classes in studio gyms around London, and I am head trainer at Ministry of Sound Fitness, which is in an old booze store in a railway arch behind the famous club's main room. It seems fitting, since I've gone from raving to behaving and training.

As a personal trainer I work with clients of all ages and abilities. But over time I have found that what really satisfies me as a coach is encouraging complete novices to lift. There are

'YOU FAIL, THEN YOU FAIL AGAIN BUT YOU KEEP GOING, KNOWING THAT ONE DAY YOU WILL ACHIEVE. AND WHEN THAT MOMENT COMES I CAN'T TELL YOU HOW SWEET IT IS.'

those people getting fit for the very first time, there are those coming back from a long period of inactivity or illness, those who want to get strong, those who want to get fit for a specific sport, and those who want a complete life transformation. It is truly an honour for me to help guide and educate people and enable them to live more productive and contented lives.

I feel I should also mention that for years I worried that I wasn't the right physique to be a personal trainer; this was possibly one of the biggest things holding me back from going for it full-time years ago. I don't look like those women on the front of women's fitness magazines. I don't have 15 per cent body fat or shredded abs. I like to be strong and celebrate what my body can do rather than worry about being super-lean or having a thigh gap. But I now know I needn't have worried; it actually made zero difference to my ability to pursue a career as a coach because being a great trainer is about so much more than what you look like. I'm not short of clients and I'm so pleased to have been involved with the #StrongIsNotASize campaign, which really resonated with me. You can be strong, and you don't have to be a specific size or shape for that to be true. For me, it was far better than the popular hashtag #strongnotskinny, which I never truly understood. It shouldn't be a choice between strong and skinny. Some people are naturally skinny, so does that mean they can't be strong as well? Being strong doesn't have a template, and we should support and empower people of all shapes and sizes to have a healthy lifestyle.

Most recently, inspired by all the incredible athletes I was fortunate enough to work and train with, I decided to compete in the sport of Strongwoman. In 2018 I entered a novice competition alongside some amazing women. This included pulling an 8-tonne bus as fast as I could over 20 metres. (That was a pretty tough one to train for – most gyms lack an 8-tonne bus to practise on!) Then there was the yoke and duck walk medley, the overhead axle, the log and circus dumbbell medley, plus loading massive stones on to platforms in the shortest time possible. If you've ever seen *Britain's Strongest Man* on the TV, you'll know the kind of thing I mean. I loved it; it's one of the best things I have ever done and the support among the competitors was unparalleled. I'm the first to admit this kind of training isn't for everyone as it is quite advanced and intense, but I have to say I've learned so much about myself by doing it and formed some incredibly powerful friendships, celebrating effort, not 'results'.

It is highly unlikely that I will ever be the world's strongest woman (I'll leave that to Donna Moore) but I love the style of training and the focus on getting stronger. Tyre flipping 180kg doesn't seem to have got boring for me yet . . .

As you can see, over the years I've experienced plenty of extremes without necessarily finding the happiness I thought I was chasing. It wasn't until I got strong in both mind and body through lifting that everything fell into place. No more fad diets, no more licking broccoli, no more juice cleanses, no more worshipping the scales – just celebrating what my body could do, surrounded by like-minded people.

So, thank you for joining me here, wherever you are in your life right now. If I have learned anything it's that striving for perfection is futile. What even is perfection? So be gentle with yourself, work with what you have and remember my mantra: 'Nothing looks as good as strong feels.'

Lifting is a man's game

Lifting will make you bulky

If you want to lose weight, cardio is better
than lifting weights

You need to go to the gym to lift

Lifting 'heavy' is the only way to get results

IT'S TIME TO BUST SOME MYTHS

There are so many myths and untruths out there about lifting weights and strength training, so before we go any further I'd like to address these head on.

1 **Lifting is a man's game** What image do you think of when someone says 'lifting weights'? I'd bet it's a muscle-bound man-hulk, all rippling abs and pecs and a cheesy grin – the kind of picture you would see on the cover of vintage weightlifting magazines from the 1960s and 1970s. But things have moved on, and lifting is absolutely no longer a man's game. Yes, historically the weights section of your average commercial gym has been a man-zone; it's where big men and me go to bicep curl. That can feel quite intimidating – not just to women, but to all beginners. In the world of personal training, we call it 'gymtimidation'.

But here's the thing. In the past couple of years I think that's really changed. We are starting to see far more women venturing into the 'man-zone' of commercial gyms because they realize that the 'toned' look (or muscle definition as I prefer to call it) they want just isn't happening for them from hours spent on the cross-trainer or treadmill or by pounding the streets for 5k. That toned look we've all been talking about for years comes from lifting weights. I think more and more women are now hearing about the amazing benefits of weight training, and it's making them rethink their workouts.

I know a lot of women who can either outlift the men or know significantly more about lifting than men. I know a lot of men who regularly train with women and I've found it's becoming less and less of a gender-specific activity. So don't let outdated stereotypes or gymtimidation put you off discovering the incredible benefits of strength training and lifting weights – for men and women.

 Lifting will make you bulky NO, NO, NO, it doesn't! Not on its own, anyway. (Can you tell I feel passionately about this one?) This myth really needs unpicking as I think it's still putting off some women doing the strength training that is beneficial for their physical and mental health.

Lifting weights on its own doesn't give you that stereotypical weightlifter's look. It builds muscle and definition, but what gives you the bulk is eating a significant calorie surplus AND lifting heavy and often.

Serious weightlifters work exceptionally hard to gain muscle bulk, and it's much harder for women to get that kind of physique even if they want to. That's partly because we have far less of the muscle-building hormone testosterone in our bodies. Even for men, who have significantly higher levels of testosterone, it takes a lot of lifting and a lot of eating to gain that kind of mass.

Take me as an example. In the past couple of years, I've been training to gain muscle size and mass for maximum strength (that's how you get to pull an 8-tonne bus). So I've been eating mostly in a calorie surplus and, yes, I guess I did become stereotypically bulky. The good news is I'm really cool with that. However, I'm also able to adapt my training to run a marathon, so being as strong as I possibly can isn't my goal for that. I'm still strong, but I'm not fuelling to grow my muscles because running is easier and quicker if you're a bit lighter. I'm still training but am eating slightly less and I'm getting closer to that lean aesthetic that I'm guessing many of you are after.

So, if your goal is to gain mass (bulk), you might do so. And if it isn't, you definitely won't. It's about understanding the link between exercise and nutrition. Oh, and if you do manage to get bulky overnight, please do tell me what you're doing because many women weightlifters out there would love to know your secret . . .

This whole debate about bulky versus lean has so many sexist overtones, anyway. Women weightlifters are often on the receiving end of sexist criticisms and body shaming comments about their muscular physique. They get comments along the lines of, 'you're looking a bit manly', or, 'careful, you don't want to be bulky', or, 'weightlifting isn't feminine'. But who says which physique is feminine? We are all in charge of our own bodies, whatever shape we are or want to be. The only thing a woman needs to be beautiful and feminine is to be herself.

If you want to lose weight, cardio is better than lifting weights If you look in the mirror and think you want to lose weight, you will obviously want to burn calories, and if you're wearing a calorie-tracker while you pound that treadmill it may well tell you that you're burning more calories during that 30 minutes on the treadmill than when you do 30 minutes of resistance training. That's true.

However, that's not the whole story: the truth is a bit more complicated. I'll talk more about this in the next chapter, but essentially, what strength training gives you is a higher percentage of lean muscle mass. That's not about being bulky, by the way, it's about having that definition. If you have more muscle mass, you'll also have a higher metabolism, so you'll burn more calories just staying alive - not just in that half an hour when you're training, but every single hour of the day and night.

So in one window of time, while you're doing cardio exercise like running or cycling, you probably will burn more calories. But it's not about just that 30-minute or one-hour snapshot: it's about the long-term lifestyle goal of achieving that functional lean-mean-machine body that feels good as well as looks good. So let's focus less on that one hour in the gym and more on the whole lifestyle. Yes, we all need cardio exercise to build our cardiovascular strength, but it's not all about doing 1,000 burpees, it's about being generally active too. A half-hour walk in your lunch break is still activity. Don't forget that intense exercise puts stress on your body, so the more you move your body in different ways and at various intensities the more benefits you'll feel in the long term.

4 **You need to go to the gym to lift** The world is your gym! If you do have access to a gym, then it can be a great experience. You've got the machines, all the facilities and access to the expertise of the people who work there. There's also the opportunity to build a community of like-minded people and it can become quite a destination – your escape, your hour of me-time away from work, the kids, the chores.

However, you don't need to splash out on a gym membership to get the benefits of strength training. You can do strength work in your living room with just a few bits of equipment. Or you can just use your own body so that your body becomes the weight. In fact, as a beginner the best place to start is to master your own body weight so that you learn the fundamentals of the key movements – the squat and the press-up, for example – before you start piling on the weights.

You can also increase the intensity of those body weight exercises. For example, I could ask you to do a squat. To increase the intensity I could ask you to do more squats in a certain time; I could give you less rest time in between sets; I could ask you to slowly lower down to the squat for 3-2-1 and ask you to hold it at the bottom so the muscle is under tension for longer and you feel that burning sensation that makes your face crease up. Believe me, that will hurt and you won't even need to be holding a weight.

If you do want to use weights, the joy of the way the fitness industry has evolved is that you can now buy them on any high street. You know those pink 3kg weights you see in Argos? They're perfect because that's 3kg more than you were working with before. There will be a time when you will outgrow them, because the more you provide a stimulus to your body the more it adapts to that stimulus. In the end, your body will become so efficient at lifting that 3kg weight that it will no longer need to use as much energy, so that particular exercise won't be as effective for you. That's why you need to keep your fitness varied, and surprise your body with new movements to grow stronger and more powerful. You certainly don't need to go to the gym to get that.

5 Lifting 'heavy' is the only way to get results

It all depends what results you're after, but in general this isn't true: you don't have to lift heavy.

Heavy is relative to the individual – what's heavy for you might not be heavy for me. It's all about the effort you're having to put in to lift that weight – I call it the RPE scale, or the Relative Perceived Exertion. As an example, doing ten air squats in a row may be an exertion level of 4 out of 10 for me. But if I asked my mum to do it, she might start struggling on the seventh one. That's a high RPE for her, so the goal for her would be to work on mastering doing those ten until it wasn't so challenging for her any more. It's only then that we might start to increase the intensity relatively. Heavy is whatever it means for the individual. You certainly don't have to lift hundreds of kilos to get a defined body; you just have to understand how to challenge yourself, progressively and safely. Lifting heavy weights when you're not used to it and haven't learned how to do it properly can be dangerous and lead to injury.

Just picking up a weight isn't all there is to strength training, anyway. There are very specific movement patterns and repetitions of those movements (reps), which I'll explain later in the book. As a rule, if you're a beginner you might start by doing a movement 8-12 times (reps). Do three or four sets of those and you should be knackered. For someone like me, who's been training for years, sometimes I will lift as heavy as I can for just five reps. That's where you progress to as you get more physically advanced, although no one should feel they have to go heavier for fewer reps if they don't want to. It's about finding a weight for you that's challenging but doesn't break you, concentrating on lifting that weight correctly so you get the right range of movement, and then building up from that point.

Sometimes people want to feel like they're progressing fast, but the truth is that the good stuff takes time. It's not a race, and don't let your ego tell you otherwise. The main thing is to get started and to enjoy the feeling of getting stronger – the results will follow. I promise you that.

2. WHY LIFT?

Women have never been encouraged to lift weights, because of the fear it would make us bulky. Rather, we've been encouraged to be 'cardio junkies', obsessed with the running machine or doing aerobics classes. I've been there, done that. For many of us, we do it not because we love it, but because we want to get thinner. It's what I call a 'transactional' approach to life, and you may recognize it in your own thought patterns. So you eat a couple of bags of crisps or have a few drinks and then think, 'God, that's at least X calories I've just guzzled my way through. Better get running!' You work out how long it might take to burn those calories, and off you go. I exhausted myself living with this mindset for years.

I get it, and in some ways that's fine – better to run off the extra calories than sit on your bum and watch Netflix all day. After all, I am an advocate of being 'active'. But if you don't love your running sessions (and I bet loads of women don't) it's kind of joyless and boring. I've watched gym-goers spend hours on the cross-trainer while mindlessly watching *EastEnders* or whatever; and really, they never look that thrilled to be doing what they are doing. I'd also question whether endless cardio torture is giving you the results you really want. I lost weight when I started serious running, but to be brutally honest, I really didn't look that great: I had no strength or 'tone' or definition, I had stick arms and in hindsight I didn't even really look all that healthy, despite what I thought the scales were telling me.

I am not knocking cardio exercise like running or walking; I do a lot of both. It is essential for our health, and we should all be doing the recommended weekly amount of 150 minutes of moderate-intensity exercise. It's just that I think lots of us have got the balance a bit wrong: all cardio and HIIT (high-intensity interval training) and no strength training.

Lifting weights is a smarter way to be stronger and if you do indeed want to look better in your clothes (as I do), then lifting will help you get there. When I first discovered lifting, it had a huge effect on my whole life outlook as well as my health. Instead of pounding the pavements – something my knees and hips didn't thank me for – I now had something I could lift. I could pick up something heavy and put it back down again. I could work on increasing the reps, increasing the amount I could hang on a bar, increasing the speed in which I could complete something. I was looking to gain – not to lose, to shrink or to take up less space on earth. I was starting to believe in myself more, and this belief was transferring to my everyday life: I had strength in my convictions, in my relationships, I was taking less s**t from people, I was standing up for myself, I was able to have a stronger position at work. My energy levels rocketed and I was sleeping well, too. I felt physically successful.

This wasn't an accident. All these benefits – and more – come from lifting weights, and it's not just me telling you this. There are now dozens and dozens of scientific studies that are providing hard, solid evidence that weight training, strength training, resistance training – whatever you want to call it – can do incredible things for you.

Let's look at what lifting weights could do for both your body and your mind, and hear from some of the people whose lives have been lifted by lifting.

You'll torch body fat

When I discovered lifting weights at CrossFit, I remember one of the first things I noticed was that I lost body fat. A lot of body fat. People were constantly telling me I looked amazing, so athletic and healthy. I lost so much weight and body fat in those first couple of months that my body didn't know what had hit it! Granted, I did go in head first and I was going four or five times a week, but the difference was incredible.

No one had ever stopped me before to tell me how good I looked, even when I was clocking up hundreds of miles of running. That's because cardio training alone doesn't give you the body composition you might be after. Yes, it will burn calories and if you are consuming fewer calories than you're using overall, you will lose weight. But where are you losing that weight from? Some of it will be fat, but some of it will be from what scientists call your 'lean body mass', which includes your muscles. So the scales may tell you that you are lighter, but you'll end up 'skinny fat', as I did. What I mean by that is you might be slim but you'll be weak, with no tone or shape (and probably aching joints from all that cardio). When you are strength training, you may not lose that much weight because you are gaining healthy muscle mass, but you will sure as hell burn fat. Which is the stuff everyone wants to lose, right?

The science is now proving what people who lift know instinctively: lifting really does torch body fat. Take this recent study on obese adults, for example.[1] All the volunteers were put on a low-calorie diet. A third of them were then given cardio workouts to do, a third were given weight-training exercises four times a week, and the other third were told not to do any exercise. So, who lost the most weight? Well, they all lost weight over the 18-month study, but the ones doing the lifting lost the most weight. That's not all. In the cardio group, a significant proportion of the weight they lost came from their lean body mass (the tissues in your body that include muscle). But the lifting group lost far more body fat, while maintaining their muscle. So, while cardio burns both fat and muscle, weightlifting burns almost exclusively fat.

And there's more good news on the fat front. Strength training may even help women, especially, burn tummy fat, which has to be good news as weight around your middle puts you at greater risk of diabetes and cardiovascular disease. Scientists gave twelve women and fourteen men a 25-week programme of resistance training, three times a week.[2] They scanned their body fat composition before and after the training, and not surprisingly both groups saw a significant reduction in body fat. But intriguingly, the women lost more fat from their bellies than the men. It was only a small study, but the same effect is seen in other research: strength training shifts tummy fat.

You'll turbo-charge your metabolism

Why is lifting is so good at burning fat? It's all about your metabolism – that's the body's biochemical processes, which transform the food you eat into useful energy (or stores it as fat if there's too much).

Your resting metabolic rate is what's important here: that's how many calories your body is using just to keep you living and breathing. Obviously if you have a higher resting metabolic rate, you burn more calories just going about your day, whether that's lounging on the sofa watching TV or even while tucked up in bed. That sounds like winning at life to me.

So, how do you raise your resting metabolic rate? The answer is, by gaining muscle. The more muscle you have, the more energy your body requires, so the more calories and fat you'll burn over a 24-hour period. In other words, having more muscle mass turns your body into a fat-burning machine, whether you're having a Sunday morning lie-in, walking the dog or sweating through one of my classes.

Research has proved that people who do weight or resistance training regularly can raise their resting metabolic rate by as much as 5–10 per cent. That could add up to burning an extra 80-plus calories a day just by living and breathing. That might not change your world in a week, but it certainly adds up over a month, a year, a lifetime.

It's not just your resting metabolic rate that's important. What's happening to your metabolism while you're working out is also crucial. Your metabolism doesn't go back to its resting level as soon as you stop exercising. It stays raised for several hours afterwards, sometimes up to 24 hours, while your body gets busy recovering from what you just put it through. This is called Excess Post-Exercise Oxygen Consumption (EPOC), or 'afterburn'. And, you've guessed it, lifting weights gives you significantly more afterburn than just doing cardio exercise, especially when you're new to it.

Case study

I have always been very active: I swam at a high level for ten years and am now a PE teacher, so I've always valued fitness. But it's only in the last couple of years that I have discovered lifting weights, and as a result I have lost 14kg, from all the right places, without weighing myself or even really trying.

I had never really got into lifting because I bought into the whole myth that lifting would make me bulky, and that doing cardio exercise would keep me looking more 'feminine'. Because of my sporting background I already had quite an athletic figure, and broad swimmer's shoulders, and I felt quite sensitive about that. I'm also quite tall, which has served me well in my sporting life, but it did make me feel as if I stuck out a little bit, something I struggled with for quite a long time.

I had been doing outdoor fitness classes for a while, and when the guy running them suggested I try lifting I was hesitant at first because of my worry about looking more manly. He assured me that wouldn't happen, so I gave it a go. I have to say I loved it from the start. Just the action of the lift makes you feel powerful and strong, and the feeling you get when you manage to lift some-thing you weren't sure you could is every bit as powerful as the 'runner's high'.

$\rightarrow$

For once I was no longer focused on my weight as a measure of my success. In fact, I stopped thinking altogether about what I weighed; my whole focus was on being stronger, and increasing how much I could lift. In September 2017 I weighed myself before the start of the new term; by the following January everyone started telling me that I had really lost weight. I said, no I don't think so, but when I weighed myself I found I had lost 7kg since the previous September. I was blown away by that as I really hadn't been trying – I was probably less worried about what I was eating than I had been in a long time. I was listening to my body, eating when I was hungry, and I wasn't afraid of carbs if I needed the energy. It was all quite intuitive.

It got to the summer and I was digging out some clothes to wear – nothing fitted me. I turned up at my mum's house and she said, 'Why are you wearing that ginormous dress?' I literally didn't have anything else that would fit. I weighed myself and discovered that I had lost another 5kg; by the time I went back to school in September I had lost 2kg more. I've stayed pretty stable since then as far as I know. I probably could have lost more, but I've gained muscle. What's interesting is that the fat has gone from all the right places, especially my stomach. I have more of a waist than I have ever had.

$\rightarrow$

As a PE teacher, I am always trying to spread the message that being strong is a fantastic goal for girls. I think a high proportion of them are still put off strength training, probably due to the old misconception that it bulks you up. We need to get to the point where women are not afraid to be strong.

I think I have a responsibility to be a role model to young women and I hope that I can continue to smash my goals so that I can tell my students about it and inspire them to join the lifting community. It's changed my life. It has helped increase my confidence and has given me opportunities to meet amazing people, and it helps relieve stress. I would encourage anyone new to lifting not to worry about what other people are thinking, lifting or doing. Focus on yourself and set yourself regular, realistic goals, then go out and train hard to beat them.

Sasha Gilbert, 29, Essex

You'll protect your bones

As far as your bones are concerned, your peak age is thirty – it's all downhill after that. Scary, right? After then our bones very slowly lose density, and for women that process really speeds up after the menopause because of the changes in our hormone levels. By the age of forty, it's estimated we're losing at least 1 per cent of bone mass every year. Obviously, that puts women at greater risk of osteoporosis, where your bones are so weak they can break even with a very minor impact.

To some extent, the rate at which you lose bone mass is genetic, which you can't do much about. Some of it is related to your diet (usually a lack of calcium, magnesium and vitamin D) but another part of it depends on your exercise levels. Taking exercise can strengthen your bones as well as your muscles. That's because when you're using a muscle, it's tugging and pushing on the bone. That stress can jolt the bone-forming cells into action. They produce more cells, and ultimately you'll have denser, stronger bones.

Research has proved that lifting weights not only maintains your bone mass and protects it against age-related decline, but it also has the power to prompt your body to build new bone. That's pretty exciting news, especially for women. One recent study of postmenopausal women with low bone mass found that just half an hour of high-intensity resistance training twice a week significantly improved their bone density and strength.[3]

You'll future-proof your muscles

Our bones aren't the only part of our bodies that decline as we age. Muscles also get weaker. This is called sarcopenia, and if you think you probably don't need to worry about that just yet, think again. We actually start losing muscle mass from about the age of thirty and if you're inactive, you could be losing between 3 and 8 per cent of your muscle mass each decade.

But muscle loss is not inevitable. Exercise will help you build muscle, and it's lifting weights that will do that most effectively. There are studies of men in their sixties and seventies who had been lifting weights for twenty years, and their muscle size and strength was identical to men forty years younger who didn't do any training.[4] It doesn't matter if you're only coming to lifting weights later in life, either. No matter what age you are, studies show you can build muscle mass by training. Even 100-year-olds can see positive changes in their muscles if they put them to good use.

Case study

Lifting isn't just for young people. I only discovered it two years ago after a lifetime of doing mindless marathons and endurance events. But what I've found is that my body has totally changed. Even though I was slim before, I had no shape, and as you get older you definitely notice that your muscle mass isn't what it was in your twenties. But now my bum is pert, my legs are toned and people are always commenting on my arms. It's got to the point where I'm happy to buy a fitted dress for a special event, whereas before I'd always choose a loose one. I never used to tuck clothes in, but now I do regularly and people comment on how good I look.

It's funny really, because I'm actually 1–2kg heavier than I used to be before lifting, but it's all about the body shape and tone. I have some old denim shorts that I only bring out for holidays and they're absolutely massive on me now. I've gone from a size 30 waist in Topshop jeans to a 28 or 26. I don't deprive myself either: I'm partial to a bit of chocolate and a glass or two of prosecco. I've found I can eat virtually anything I want and don't change size, which is probably down to the fact that when you lift your body continues to burn calories for hours afterwards.

$\rightarrow$

I used to be obsessed with the scales but the only time I weigh myself now is to check which weight I need to choose when I want to lift my own body weight. It's fair to say I've really got into lifting. What I'm currently aiming for is to be able to lift double my body weight, and I'm about 6kg away from that goal at the moment. That's something I would never have dreamed I could do, even in my twenties.

Lifting has really lifted my confidence. That's partly down to better body confidence, but I think it's also because you're always setting yourself little goals, and when you achieve them you feel pretty great afterwards. I'm constantly trying to improve, and I stay accountable to myself by writing down my targets or putting them on Instagram. There's nothing like stating your intentions on social media for making you stick to them!

Another reason it has helped is that I train with other people in a supportive atmosphere, which is a real boost to my confidence, even though most of them are much younger than me. I don't try to compete with them but I have to admit it gives me a bit of satisfaction when I'm lifting heavier than them.

Clare Shepherd, 44, Hertfordshire

You'll improve your posture

Modern life is officially terrible for our posture. Just think of the way we all sit hunched over our desks at work for hours on end, and then come home and lounge on the sofa. All this prolonged sitting puts strain on our back, our hamstrings (the muscles at the back of the thighs) and our neck and shoulders, and it causes those all-important gluteal muscles in our bottoms to wither away. No wonder sitting is being called the new smoking. Then, when we do stand up, our neck and shoulders hunch forwards and our spines are rounded in a 'C' shape rather than the natural 'S' curve they should have.

Lifting weights can help to offset that damage to your posture by strengthening the muscles that support you when you're sitting, standing or just doing all those movements that are part of normal life – whether that's carrying your shopping bags, reaching a high cupboard or running after your toddler who has just decided to leg it out of the door of the supermarket. How many times have you heard of someone putting their back out just by picking their keys up from the floor? That's not to say that training will prevent any injuries from happening, but it will ensure you are less susceptible to them.

We know that strength training reduces the risk of injury, not only because it builds muscle, but because it also strengthens ligaments, tendons and joint cartilage. And this will encourage you to stand tall and proud with your shoulders back, and it also improves your balance, which is pretty important as you get older. Lots of research has pointed out how important resistance training is for the elderly so they can reduce their risk of falls. You see, you're never too old to start lifting!

You'll be happier

We hear a lot about how exercise can improve your mental health, and there's plenty of evidence to back this up. What happens when we exercise is that our bodies release chemicals that can make us feel calmer and happier. You've probably heard of endorphins, the neurotransmitters released by the brain that give us that 'runner's high' feeling. But there are other feel-good chemicals that are unlocked by exercise, such as serotonin and dopamine, which all play a part in regulating our mood. No wonder exercise is officially sanctioned as a treatment for mild to moderate depression by the National Institute for Health and Care Excellence in the UK.[5]

However, most of the research so far has been done on cardio exercise, usually walking or jogging, and there hasn't been as much information about what strength training or lifting weights can do for your mental health. But a big new study published in 2018[6] concluded that resistance training had a huge impact on how depressed people felt. It didn't seem to matter whether they did it every day or a couple of times a week, or even how healthy they were to start with. In fact, the scientists found it didn't even matter if people got stronger or not – just doing the training was enough to lift their spirits.

Interestingly, those feeling the most down saw the biggest improvements to their mood. That's great news for people in the early stages of depression or those who have hit a tough point in life. Weight training really does have the power to help lift that fog, and I can certainly relate to this. When I trained in the morning before work, or even if I was still on a high from the previous evening's gym session, it genuinely made me more optimistic at work and in life. I was more able to find solutions to challenging situations and was calmer in my approach.

Other studies have proved that lifting weights can reduce feelings of anxiety and make you feel calmer. In studies, women especially have reported feeling far less anxious after just one weight training session, which is pretty remarkable.

Not only that, but lifting improves self-esteem and body image. One study which pitted yoga against strength training[7] discovered that both groups improved their mental health and felt less depressed, but the ones lifting also had a more positive body image than the yogis. And a small study of young women that tested the benefits of weight training against running found that it was the lifters who significantly improved their self-esteem.

Case study

I never planned to get into lifting. I just tried out a decent-looking new gym and really enjoyed the lifting sessions. I felt really great after them and I was pretty good at it – I didn't expect that. Before I started, a bunch of things crossed my mind about lifting: I wasn't strong enough, I'm not dedicated enough, I party too much to keep it up (sorry mum), I'll end up super-bulky. But I stuck at it because the coaches made me feel great and I left the classes feeling awesome.

When I was younger I suffered from depression, and a couple of years ago I started suffering really badly from anxiety. Sometimes I struggled to get out of bed and get to work, and eventually I had to take some time off. I knew from experience that exercise was a really effective treatment for depression, but the thought of getting to the gym before work was just so difficult; a good day was when I managed to get myself up and into the office by 10am.

I started doing Laura's LIFTED classes at Ministry of Sound Fitness once a week on a Tuesday evening, plus another lifting class if I could make it, and I have to say they made a massive difference to my mental health. What I find about lifting is that you feel so positive when you manage it: you feel you have really achieved something. That sense of physical strength makes you feel mentally

→

strong, too, and you leave the gym with a swagger that really spreads into the rest of your life. You feel you can take on the world, and things that seemed daunting before now look do-able. It's also an escape from the real world, 45 minutes where I can lose myself and my anxiety and put all my focus into trying to lift, in a trusted place with awesome coaches who really care about my wellbeing. Nothing else matters while I'm in those sessions (apart from Shazam-ing the TUNES!) and I feel like I can be the best version of myself for a while.

I have already achieved my lifting goal for this year, which was to deadlift 100kg. It has taken me a year of training once or twice a week to get to that point, but when I started I never ever thought I would actually do it. It's given me such a buzz.

However, that's not to say that lifting is some miracle cure for anxiety and depression. Recently, I have been struggling a bit again, and there have been times when I have missed sessions and been unable to work. But I try really hard to get back to my lifting classes because I know that when I do, I feel better afterwards – the next day I notice a definite improvement in my mood and wellbeing.

I would say to anyone thinking of starting to lift, particularly if you're not in a great place in your head: everyone has to start somewhere, and it really helps to find the most welcoming gym and helpful coach, as I did, and go from there.

Jen Armstrong-McKay, 33, London

You'll feel more confident

The thing about lifting is that you're constantly challenging yourself. Can I lift this today? I couldn't do it yesterday, but how about today? You start with small goals, but over the weeks you'll visibly see and feel yourself getting stronger. Soon you'll be doing things you never thought you'd be able to – and that does amazing things for your confidence levels. There's nothing quite like feeling strong: it's totally empowering, and that trickles into every area of your life.

Setting goals and continuously challenging yourself gives you that feeling of power and control: you're in charge of your training. That can't help but give you a huge boost of self-confidence.

Then there's the social aspect of lifting. You won't get this if you choose to work out at home, but if you do join a class or a gym, one thing you'll notice pretty soon is that lifters are a fantastic and supportive community. This social support is really beneficial, as not only does it help you stick to the training, it also gives you better life satisfaction.

I regularly witness the development of confidence and mental strength through my gym community. It gives you a sense of purpose, a sense of belonging – almost to the extent that if you didn't turn up, you would be doing an injustice to yourself and the gang. Gyms have their own special energy, and when you find a community that suits you and your goals, it is hugely empowering, because no matter where you are at, people will cheer you on until the very last rep.

You'll have more energy

You'd think exercise would make you tired because it's using up your energy, but the opposite happens. Research has proved that upping your activity levels makes you less tired in day-to-day life and in fact gives you more get-up-and-go, not less.

Exactly why this is isn't clear, but scientists think it's probably down to those 'happy' chemicals in your brain, which are released when you exercise. Neurotransmitters like dopamine, serotonin and norepinephrine play a part in boosting your mood and can also help you feel more energized. It could also be because lifting weights is giving you better strength and endurance, which helps you get through the day without getting so tired. Or it might be because it improves your sleep, in terms of both quantity and quality. My clients tell me they've never slept as well since taking up lifting and this is backed up by research, this time among older men, which showed that just 12 weeks of regular resistance training helped them wake up less often and sleep better at night.[8]

Case study

I was a true cardio girl, or so I thought. But after several years of running marathons, it got to the stage where running was no longer doing a huge amount for me. I didn't seem to be getting any fitter, and I certainly wasn't getting the muscle tone I was after. I wasn't exactly bored, but I needed another challenge, something to really boost my energy levels.

So I signed up with a personal trainer, who introduced me to strength training. At first we did circuits-type workouts in the park, doing body weight exercises or using really basic equipment like kettlebells or whatever was around us, like park benches or playground equipment. But then winter came along and she suggested we try the local gym. It was a real strongman-type gym, full of men lifting impossibly heavy weights – not the sort of place I'd ever have walked into on my own. But I enjoyed it so much more than I thought I would, and all feelings of intimidation passed. She taught me all the basics of using free weights, and very quickly I noticed my strength and energy levels improve.

The more I did it, the more I wanted to do it. I was getting the same high from achieving a new one rep max record (the maximum amount you

→

can lift for one repetition) as I had been getting from a new personal best on a run. But the difference was that I found the act of lifting weights so much more satisfying than running for miles. With lifting weights, every single session gives you that 'wow' feeling, that feeling of accomplishment. It's really helped take my fitness to a new level, to tone up more effectively, become stronger and ultimately more confident.

I take back everything I ever said about not being a weights girl: I'm a complete convert. I'm still running, but I also make sure I lift about three times a week to get a really nice balance.

These days, if anyone asks me for advice on how to lose weight, tone up or get fitter, I always recommend weight training. Cardio is definitely still essential but I've found it just doesn't work on its own. If you don't have the confidence to head straight to the weights section of a gym or join a class, work with a personal trainer for a few sessions; this will enable you to build up your confidence in a safe, more private space before branching out on your own.

Michelle Stoodley, 33, London

You'll deal with stress better

There's really nothing like lifting weights for bringing down your stress levels. Some of my clients have extremely stressful jobs and they tell me that the hour they spend with me is the best stress reliever of the whole day. With a lot of the evening sessions I coach, I see people walk in with stressed faces and tense shoulders, talking on their phones, about a 'mad' day. Then slowly through the session, their focus shifts to their physical performance and they forget about whatever was on their mind. They leave with a different perspective than when they arrived, and it's wonderful to see. I think it's because of what you're physically doing when you're lifting: the power and exertion of the movement allows you to release all that pent-up emotional and physical stress. It's as if you're channelling your stress directly into that weight.

Scientists have looked at what happens to people's stress hormone levels when they give them something nerve-racking to do. Volunteers are asked to prepare a five-minute public speaking presentation – but their notes are taken away from them just before they are due to speak. In one study, men who were used to lifting weights were given this test alongside men who had never lifted weights. Not surprisingly, levels of the stress hormone cortisol shot up in both groups. But what happened to their heart rate was interesting: the hearts of the non-exercisers raced, whereas the heart rate of the lifters stayed pretty stable. The researchers concluded that lifting weights had helped those men deal more effectively with stress.

Case study

Fitness has become a large part of my life over the last two years. I have not only lost weight but have gained confidence, dealt with stress better, enjoyed new experiences and made memories and strong friendships. It has also improved my mental health by giving me something to focus on outside of my work life. Lifting in particular has been a great way to push myself, getting physically stronger and proving to myself and my doubters that I am worth more and can do better.

Strength to me means overcoming your past and not allowing what has happened before to ruin or rule your life. I will admit this is something I still struggle with at times, but fitness is giving me an outlet for my stress, anxiety and feelings of loneliness. Because of regular exercise I am the most physically strong and the fittest I have been in my adult life. I am still a beginner to lifting but I am enjoying all the new challenges. Strength can be a powerful thing; it can empower people, especially women, to accomplish things they only dreamed about before.

Nicola Chamberlain, 33, Hertford

You'll have a healthier heart

There is no question that cardio exercise is good for your heart – the clue's in the name. But it has now been proved that lifting can have the same benefits for your cardiovascular system. Weight training has a positive impact on at least three aspects of heart health: blood pressure, cholesterol and blood sugar control.

When a study examined what was happening inside people's bodies following 45 minutes of moderate-intensity resistance training at the gym, it was discovered that the training reduced their blood pressure by up to 20 per cent, which the researchers said was better than taking medication for high blood pressure.[9] Not only that, but the benefits continued for half an hour afterwards, and for people who trained for 30–45 minutes three times a week, their blood pressure stayed low for twenty-four hours after training ended. Having high blood pressure can lead to heart attacks and strokes and it's a pretty common problem as we get older, so it's clear that lifting weights could help you keep yours under control.

Having high cholesterol can also lead you towards heart problems in later life. The evidence here is a bit more mixed, but some studies have found that weight training can cut the 'bad' cholesterol in your body, while increasing the 'good' cholesterol that protects your heart.

You remember how we naturally lose muscle mass as we age (unless we train to keep it, of course)? For complicated biochemical reasons, that puts you more at risk of getting type 2 diabetes as you get older, particularly if you're inactive and put on weight around your middle. So if you're building muscle as you age rather than losing it, it's going to play a big part in helping to control your blood sugar levels. If you already have type 2 diabetes, there's further good news. One study found that two sessions a week of weight training that gets gradually more challenging can improve insulin sensitivity and blood sugar levels, as well as reduce tummy fat – and that was without any changes to the volunteers' diet.[10]

You'll think more clearly

So many people tell me that they are able to be more productive at work after a lifting session. It seems to lift that brain fog and help you focus your mind for the day ahead.

Scientists aren't really sure why it happens, but exercise really does appear to super-charge your brainpower and alertness. They think maybe it's because it's pumping more blood to your brain. Or it could be because you sleep better. There are even some studies that suggest that exercise might be able to prompt your brain to create new brain cells. Now that's what I call a benefit!

Lifting weights may even make you cleverer and keep your brain sharp as you age. Research among older people who were having trouble with their memory discovered that those who did resistance exercises twice a week for six months increased their physical strength.[11] And incredibly, as they got stronger their cognitive powers got stronger as well. Best of all, the benefits persisted even a year after the experiment, with scans showing that they actually increased the size of their grey matter! Meanwhile, the volunteers just doing stretching exercises didn't have any improvements in their memories or brainpower. Other studies have found similar results: neither walking nor balance exercises have as big an effect on the brain as resistance workouts.

Case study

Strength to me means both physical and mental strength. Strength is not a particular number or phrase, it's putting 100 per cent into everything you do and feeling 'grounded' in what you do. I got into lifting by going to a free women's lifting taster session at my local gym. I had an amazing time, and managed to find a personal trainer who loves to lift and is brilliant at helping me with my self-confidence. Through lifting I have gained so much confidence and self-belief in all areas of my life. I also lost one and a half stone through training, meaning I feel lighter, less sluggish and more alert.

I now don't really worry or get anxious about life changes or doing something new. I have also met so many like-minded people and am part of a friendly community who are always ready to help anyone out.

I advise all first timers to just go for it. See if there are any free taster sessions around, or take a friend along to a class. Anything you do, however small, will help you reach your goals. Also, ask around if you aren't sure about anything, and you'll be surprised at the amount of people who are willing to help you out.

Emily Mulkerrin, 28, West Yorkshire

You MIGHT even live longer

Sadly I can't promise you eternal life (I wish I could!) but there's now a lot of evidence building up to show that lifting weights could help you live a longer life as well as a healthier one.

A massive study of 80,000 British people carried out over a nine-year period[12] found that two sessions a week of body weight exercises like sit-ups, push-ups or lifting weights reduced the risk of premature death by more than 20 per cent. It also cut down the risk of dying of cancer by an amazing 31 per cent. Cardio exercise was also found to reduce the risk of dying early, but it had zero effect on the risk of dying from cancer. Now as someone with a lot of cancer in my family, I think that's a pretty extraordinary finding. We don't yet understand why building up muscle and strength could have that kind of effect on your body. But to me, that's one pretty compelling reason to get lifting!

3. MY TEN COMMANDMENTS FOR LIFTING . . . AND FOR LIFE

1. Thou shalt . . . start somewhere

2. Thou shalt not . . . train for a thigh gap

3. Thou shalt . . . do it for the feeling

4. Thou shalt . . . focus on form

5. Thou shalt . . . fuel your body for its function

6. Thou shalt . . . never compare your journey

7. Thou shalt . . . keep going when the going gets tough (because it will)

8. Thou shalt . . . swerve the bulls**t

9. Thou shalt . . . rest and recover

10. Thou shalt . . . respect the process

Now you know that lifting can benefit your physical and mental health in so many amazing ways, you are probably raring to go and, er, lift something. That's fantastic, but before you rush off and try to deadlift your own body weight, you need a proper plan. Just like in life, in lifting there are no quick fixes, no miracle solutions, no magic potions (and certainly no detox tea) to drink. There is hard work and commitment ahead, but so many gains and rewards to be made.

Here are my ten commandments so you can truly lift yourself.

1. Thou shalt . . . start somewhere

For most of my life, I've said to myself, 'I'll be happy when . . .' This mainly revolved around my weight, as you know, but in doing that I think I created this sense of self-sabotage and weird self-loathing. The reality is, I just didn't know what I had to do to make a change.

When I look back, I realize that every 'start' I made was really extreme. It usually involved some kind of calorie restriction, as well as committing myself to huge amounts of exercise or some ridiculous challenge that seemed like a lot to fit into my already busy life.

Here's a fantastic example of one of my many 'starts' – maybe you can relate to this: 'So, on Monday I am going to start a 30-day challenge. I am going to go to the gym three times a week after work, I am going to run 5k three times a week, and I am going to follow the 5:2 diet.' The 5:2 diet, for those fortunate enough never to have tried it, means you eat normally five days a week, and for two days a week you eat just 500 calories. Who can survive on 500 calories? My minimum energy requirement is about 2,000 calories a day, so this was a huge deficit, which was mentally and physically challenging. Ask me how pumped I was to go to Body Pump at Virgin Active Hammersmith the next day? (Yes I did this before I found CrossFit.) I wasn't. Not one bit. I was cursing the unbelievably chirpy instructor at 6am telling me to give 110 per cent (which really annoys me as that's technically impossible). I couldn't because I had absolutely zero energy. It was a very all-or-nothing approach, and that's me all over. If I commit to doing something, I genuinely try to give it everything, but how long can I give my everything to something that ultimately is not sustainable while living a normal life? I'd fall off, I'd beat myself up and the cycle would continue.

So when I say 'start somewhere' I don't mean do it how I did it. A good place to start is to assess where you are at right now. You could start by writing yourself a little bio – how would you describe yourself in a paragraph? Consider the following:

How do I feel about myself now?

Am I satisfied with my current lifestyle?

How much sleep do I get per night?

Am I paying attention to my stress and am I managing it well?

Am I happy with what I'm eating?

Am I satisfied with my current activity levels?

Who are my role models?

Am I surrounded by supporters?

What are my goals?

Am I achieving them?

I can't stress enough how important it is to find a fitness activity you are passionate about. It could be that you absolutely love doing home workouts when your little one takes a nap; it could be that CrossFit is totally your vibe; or you could decide that group HIIT (high-intensity interval training) and circuit training or maybe dance fitness will ignite your fire. Whatever it is, DO THAT. Make time for it. You don't have to be great to start, but you do have to start to be great.

Here are my dos and don'ts for getting started:

- Don't do as I did and promise yourself you're going to do that class or that home workout a silly number of times a day. Keep it real. Decide on what type of training you want to do and when, and how it is going to fit into your weekly schedule. Start small and build on your success.

- Do surround yourself with genuine people who are supportive of you and your goals. It's even better if you can train with a friend, whether that's in your living room, at a gym class or in the park. One good way to get started is to get a gang together and share the cost of a personal trainer for however long you can afford. That way, you'll get the expert attention to make sure you're lifting and working correctly, and have a well-balanced programme to suit your body.

- Don't expect too much of yourself too early on. Just set yourself an initial goal to turn up at the session, and give it your best. I think one of my problems with all those false starts was that I was expecting to see change too quickly. Seven days to rock-solid abs? No. Whatever you've read on Instagram, that's not going to happen. Despite what the waist training enthusiasts try to tell you.

- Do know that not every day is going to feel like an awesome training day. It's going to be tough some days and you may not always feel motivated, but ensure you maintain discipline so you can form a habit that becomes part of your lifestyle. So on the days when you really feel like turning up, go for it, and on the days when you don't feel like turning up, just make sure you turn up! (Unless of course you are unwell . . . that's obviously different.)

- Don't fall into the 'I'll start after the New Year' or 'I'll start when the kids go back to school' trap. Just start and don't look back. Decide on a goal, keep it small, keep it simple and commit to putting effort into it.

2. Thou shalt not . . . train for a thigh gap

When you're training you need a goal, a focus, something to keep in mind when the going gets tough. But how do you know when it's the wrong one? Well, mine was always to lose weight, to get a thigh gap – basically to shrink myself. The trouble with having weight loss as your goal is that it just doesn't really work, if we are honest, otherwise we would all be size 8s by now. There seem to be too many ways to fail when you make weight loss your goal. You try to 'be good' with your diet, then before you know it you are raiding the fridge for chocolate or leftovers from dinner at 10pm out of sheer gnawing hunger, temptation or because of a million complicated reasons we probably can't even admit to ourselves (trust me, I had a bad and ill-informed relationship with food for years). Then because we've 'given in' and 'failed' we just give up, and so the next diet can wait until next Monday. Sound like a familiar cycle? I think this happens because when you have losing weight as your goal, you are focusing on self-deprivation. It's dull, it's soulless, it's negative . . . and ultimately really, really difficult to achieve.

When I finally realized I had been focusing on all the wrong goals for most of my life, I knew I had to set some new ones. Yes, I wanted to look better, fit into my clothes better, and worry less about myself naked. But did that have to mean I had to focus all my energies on losing weight? No. When I discovered working with weights at CrossFit, for the first time I had a goal that didn't revolve around what my scales said each week. I just wanted to get better at it, and focus all my energy on perfecting the movements and building my strength. I started to love how strong it made me feel, both physically and mentally. I was no longer so bothered about what I weighed; my goal was on my strength and fitness. I was proud of my body and what it could do, not ashamed of how it looked. That was a huge change in mindset for me. So my advice would be, don't do it for the thigh gap, do it to be strong and fit. It's incredibly liberating.

Of course, our goals can change over time. My goal is still to be as strong as I possibly can, but I am currently training for a marathon so ideally I need to be a bit lighter to make it easier to run long distance. That has meant I've had to cut down on my calorie intake but I haven't gone mad with it – no more crazy juice cleanses or inhaling kale from a tiny mug! As I write this I am about halfway through running a small daily 'calorie deficit', meaning that I'm taking in fewer calories per day than I'm using. I'm still strength training though, as having a strong core and strong glutes and hamstrings gives you power as a runner. But I recognize that it might be harder to lift as heavy and as often as I was when I was fuelling for strength gains and I've had to adapt my goals accordingly.

I need you to know that good change takes time and having an unrealistic short-term goal may just get you down. So, set yourself a long-term goal, like getting strong, and then break it down into manageable chunks, or 'micro' goals. So these could be:

- Managing two 30-minute strength training sessions a week

- Getting out in your lunch break or after work twice a week for a brisk 20- or 30-minute walk

You can build up those micro goals as the weeks go on; just keep it realistic and tick it off when you've managed to ace it. When you have actual, tangible goals like this you take the focus off your weight and on to the functional things your body can do. This journey isn't linear and the results aren't always predictable – science, your genetics and life in general all play a part! But if you are focusing on consistently doing the right things for your goals, you WILL see results in time. The rest – weight loss, fat loss – comes as a by-product of having a fit body. Get strong and the rest will follow.

And my advice for achieving a thigh gap? Just stand with your legs apart a little bit. That should do it.

3. Thou shalt . . . do it for the feeling

'If I do this class, will I end up getting big? Because I don't want to look like you.' This was an actual thing someone said to me once. If they had said that to me five years ago I probably would have cried in the bathroom, gone on a downward mental spiral and fallen out of a good routine. I am so grateful now that I am happy in my own skin that this kind of comment doesn't bother me; in fact, I find it fascinating. Who says what a woman's body 'should' look like? Are these rules written down in some secret book somewhere? I feel sorry that this person was trapped by her own aesthetic ideals. I can't remember now exactly how I replied, but the reality is, it has taken me years to get to this point with my strength, and a one-hour training session isn't going to turn you into me overnight.

Comments like that make you realize how we judge other people's bodies all the time, whether consciously or subconsciously. I have been on the receiving end of a lot of judgement, comparison and commentary on my size and shape. I am not offended by this one bit as my body now has a purpose: it can do cool stuff like lift heavy weights and pull an 8-tonne bus; I have good posture; and lifting has given me real mental clarity and focus.

I think that's because when you lift, you can't think about anything else. You have to focus 100 per cent on the movement and get the technique right; there's no room in your mind for worrying about work deadlines, chores or office politics. Each time you practise a move, you should be thinking about how your body feels at every point of the lift. I say to my clients, take your mind to the muscle as you lift, and squeeze physically AND mentally. Developing that mind–muscle connection is really important. To me, the act of lifting is almost like meditating – that moment of calm focus where you empty your mind of all the other stuff bothering you and put your everything into the lift. It's that one hour of the day when nothing else matters. Whatever your other priorities and deadlines, you set that one hour aside and try your best. The great strength coach Charles Poliquin once said 'celebrate effort not results'. I love that.

There will be days you turn up to the bar and find you're not very good, but on other days you will be amazing. It's important to realize that your progress will not always be linear, but when you have been practising a lift and finally achieve it, the feeling of euphoria is quite incredible. You feel anything is possible, not just in the gym but in life. I remember a time when the strongman log at my gym was completely beyond me to press. The yellow one (it's most people's nemesis as it's just a little bit heavy and awkward). I just couldn't do it. I wasn't strong enough, so I tried and tried and tried until it went up (so many fails!). Now, one year on, it feels easy. It was a good lesson in how when the good stuff comes, it really means something. Lifting is my therapy and a lot of my friendship group feel the same about lifting, too.

I think weightlifting teaches you a lot about life: in order to succeed, you have to master the basics, then develop slowly, with a lot of misses and fails along the way. You pick yourself up after the fails and try, try again. You reflect on what went wrong and learn from it. And when you finally make that lift, you can do anything. Really, anything.

4. Thou shalt . . . focus on form

If you are a total beginner, let me first say, congratulations! You have decided to start resistance training to bulletproof your body. Having a strong, fit and healthy body will transfer energy and positivity into the rest of your life, I have no doubt.

But getting started can appear a little daunting, so just know that form and technique is more important than intensity. It's really important to make sure you nail the movement patterns before you start piling the weight on. That's why I always advise beginners to consult a fitness professional if they can: take up one of those free trial offers for a personal trainer at the gym, or get together with friends to hire one. If that isn't possible, perhaps find a strength training plan that works for you to do at home, and mix it up with some group lifting classes or an outdoor boot camp so you have some support from a professional in nailing your form. Lifting with poor technique, in other words if someone has not been taught correctly, is something we see a lot and this can lead to injury.

It is best to start learning certain movements with no weights at all, just using your body weight. That way, you will be able to focus on your technique, perfect the movement pattern and work out your current strength and range of motion. What I mean by range of motion is how far your body can take a certain movement, in other words the full movement potential at a joint, or flexion or extension. So, imagine a squat. You've probably heard of the phrase 'ass to grass', and although that's going to be pretty impossible for most of us, the ideal is to get your bum lower than parallel to your knees. Everyone's range is going to be different, depending on their experience and their mobility, which in turn depends a lot on how they are built and their sporting history. But it's super-important to find the correct position so you can get low enough in the squat to use the full movement range at the joint. Every time you practise a squat you are trying to get a fuller range of movement, potentially breaking down the fascia (the connective tissue) in the muscle to hit better depth, which will in turn improve the results. There's no point in doing half a squat 20 times; better to concentrate on doing five with really good form. Don't even think about adding weights to that movement until you've truly mastered it.

Once you get started, there can be a lot of pressure to feel like you need to make fast progress and lift heavier weights but this isn't the right way to go about it. There are many different ways of increasing the intensity of your move: you can do more reps, more sets, change the tempo, or cut down your rest time in between sets. That's all without adding any more weight. It is important to ensure you are not working more quickly than your body can cope with and stressing it unnecessarily; your body needs time to adapt to the new stimulus. Just because Mobility Mandy or Strong Sally next to you is squatting with the 12kg weight, it doesn't mean you have to. Build strong movement patterns, get confident in the range and then you can start to extend yourself. In the professional world, we call this 'progressive overload', where you very gradually increase the demands on your muscles, which stimulates those muscles to grow. It is far more important to get the lift right and start small than go for heavy weights or high reps early on. It's not a race.

As a beginner it is important to find a weight that challenges you but doesn't pull you out of poor form to complete. Always start small if you're new to lifting: a 3kg or 4kg dumbbell might be about right if you are a complete newbie. But again, depending on your physical and sporting history, you may naturally be able to control load well already, so find what feels challenging to you.

How you breathe is another important aspect of your form. While it may be tempting to hold your breath during a movement, the best way to breathe during resistance training is to inhale as you lower the weight and exhale as you lift the weight. This helps to control your blood pressure while lifting, and also supports the spine, protecting it from injury and helping it to stay stable. (I will talk more about how heavy your weights should be and how to breathe correctly in the next chapter.)

As you pursue your strength training journey, you might find it helpful to video your session on your phone so you can check back on your form. It can be a real eye-opener to see what the lift looked like in reality versus how it felt. You are your own personal trainer! I film mine all the time; it's amazing to look back and see how far you have come.

5. Thou shalt . . . fuel your body for its function

When I look back at what I used to eat, I'm embarrassed. Honestly, I used to go to CrossFit, train hard and then eat a load of pineapple. Now, in one sense there's nothing wrong with pineapple. Fruit equals health, right? But in this context I needed to ask these questions:

- what nutritional value does it have?

- where is the protein that would aid my post-workout recovery?

- exactly how many calories was I taking in from soft fruit that was high in natural sugars?

This approach to nutrition wasn't rational, and it wasn't educated. I needed to learn what my body needed, and what it could handle in order to lose fat sustainably and still train. What I learned was that eating a massive packet of cashews isn't actually very ideal for fat loss either. As nice as a cashew is, there are HUGE amounts of calories in nuts. (Nuts are a good, healthy food, by the way, just not in the quantities I was eating them.) And eating an omelette and a couple of jelly babies offered from my mate Katherine probably wasn't going to help either. I needed to understand what my body needed to fuel my training, and a plan for how to get there, without feeling like I was restricting myself unnecessarily.

So, let's talk about the energy balance equation. That is, energy in versus energy out. At a very basic level, if your energy out is consistently more than your energy in, then you will very likely lose fat. If energy in is higher than energy out, you are likely to gain fat. It's really that simple. It doesn't matter how hard you train; if you are not eating well, you are not going to be working at your true potential. For optimal performance you should be consuming a good range of the three main macronutrients, and keeping your protein levels high in particular. These macronutrients are:

- **Protein** An essential part of our diets, protein is involved in almost all our bodily processes. It is vital for building and repairing tissue, hormone production, plus skin, hair and bone health. Most importantly from a lifting point of view, it provides the body with amino acids, which are the building blocks of muscle. Eating lean sources of protein such as white fish, turkey, salmon, venison, chicken, pork and eggs, as well as plant-based proteins such as chickpeas, beans and lentils, provides a great foundation for a well-balanced diet.

- **Carbohydrates** Demonized by so many, carbs are a vital part of a balanced diet. They are the body's primary source of energy and provide fuel for our brains. When most people think of carbs they think of bread and pasta. But it's complex carbohydrates that will give you sustained energy: think brown rice, sweet potatoes, whole grains, nuts, seeds and vegetables. Cutting down sugary 'simple carbs' like cakes, biscuits, white bread and fizzy drinks can really help if your goal is fat loss. But beware: zero-carb diets are not a good idea. They will make you feel like you are swimming through treacle when you are strength training.

- **Fat** Again, fat gets a bad press. But fat is essential for a healthy diet. Aim for the good types of fat (monounsaturated and polyunsaturated fats), which are present in foods such as avocados, nuts, seeds, salmon, tuna and mackerel.

Providing your body with a balance of the above macro-nutrients plus good amounts of vegetables (especially green, leafy ones) will also ensure that you are getting the micro-nutrients (vitamins and minerals) you need to maintain optimum health, strong bones, healthy skin and a strong immune system.

A word on protein

People often ask me if they need to be eating a lot more protein now that they have started strength training, because they've heard that it's protein that fuels the growth of muscle tissue. My answer is, yes, a diet high in protein will definitely help you build muscle mass and recover well from your training. But the question of how much protein you need is more complicated, because it depends on your goals. If I'm training for a Strongwoman competition, I'm going to need more protein than you will if you're a newbie doing three 30-minute strength training sessions a week. It also depends on your weight. As a guide, the Department of Health recommends about 0.75g of protein per kilo of body weight, so that's about 50g of protein a day for someone who is 64kg (10 stone) (see page 103). However, there are a lot of arguments in scientific circles about whether that's too low, especially for people who are trying to lose weight. That's because when we're cutting calories to lose weight, we also tend to lose muscle mass. So eating extra protein can help keep your muscles topped up. Some studies have shown that dieters should eat 1.6g of protein per kilo of body weight, which would be more like 102g a day for a 64kg person. Essentially, you have to decide what works for you, depending on your goals.

People often worry about when and how they should eat: should they eat loads of protein after training to help muscle repair and growth? Should they carb-load before a session to give them more energy? My answer is that it's more important to look at the bigger picture of what you are eating over a day, and over a week. If you make sure your diet is balanced, that it contains the three macronutrients above plus lots of vegetables, it doesn't really matter what you eat when. Sure, if you like to eat a banana half an hour before a session because you think it gives you an energy buzz, then go for it. Although I have to say that, biologically speaking, a banana 30 minutes before a workout is pretty unlikely to give you energy because your body won't have had time to digest it, and I would generally advise against eating one to two hours before a session because it can make you feel sick during exercise. But if that banana makes you feel good, then go ahead – eat it. Or if you feel that a high-protein snack like a peanut butter smoothie right after a workout makes you feel good, do that too if it fits in with your overall intake of nutrients that day. But you certainly don't have to eat protein after a workout. There are no hard and fast rules and there is a danger of over-complicating these things. Do what feels right for you and remember the bigger picture: that energy-in, energy-out balance.

6. Thou shalt . . . never compare your journey

It's incredibly tempting to look at someone else and say, 'I'm not a strong as . . .', 'I'm not as thin as . . .', 'I'm not as good as . . .' Realizing that one size does not fit all was really my 'aha' moment. I could either spend my life trying to be like someone else, or I could work with what I had and play to my strengths – quite literally! This is probably one of the hardest lessons to learn when you are new to this game.

Focus on getting your own s**t done, go at your own pace, and understand that no one is looking at you when you're training in a class or in the gym. Really. They are all too busy thinking about themselves.

Monitoring your progress is a really good way to track the journey. It can be super-motivating to see and feel the results, whether that's how your clothes fit, how you're performing in your training sessions or changes in your daily energy levels. If you find a method of tracking you like, stick with that. There is no right or wrong here. Here are some ways you can track your progress:

- Take a photo of yourself (in underwear if you're brave) every four weeks. Try to ensure you take it at the same time of day, with the same lighting and outfit. Over time, change will be very visible.

- Body composition analysis. This uses a machine or callipers to measure body fat and muscle mass. You will probably be able to do this at your local gym: it's a great way of managing your goals that doesn't revolve around the scales.

- Weigh yourself. You know by now that I personally don't do this. But if it's your preferred method, then okay, as long as you do it at the same time every week or month for a consistent, accurate assessment. It is important to remember that the scales are not always an accurate representation of progress. There are so many reasons why your weight may fluctuate day to day and week to week: water retention, salt intake, hormone levels (especially for women), stress, exposure to heat, a change in dietary fibre levels and . . . you gained muscle! The scales do not tell the whole story.

'DON'T COMPARE THE SPEED OF YOUR PROGRESS TO ANYONE ELSE'S; THEY ARE NOT YOU. JUST DO YOU!'

Don't worry about the day-to-day changes; look at the trend, from the start to the current day, and stick with it for at least 30 days. If things aren't going in the right direction, reassess and change something.

- Measure yourself. Use a tape measure around your waist (at about belly button level) and hips (the widest point around your rear) every four weeks.

Personally, I prefer the photo option. It's super-easy, is personal to you and is a useful way to monitor your progress in the medium term. Just don't do it every day or even every week, otherwise you'll be chasing daily goals that don't mean much. It's more important to focus on the medium term. I would always use the rule that it takes four weeks of sticking to your plan consistently to see any real change in your shape. You may experience results before this point, but if you don't, don't get deflated; everyone is different.

So the message is, stick with it for the long haul and fall in love with the *process* right now, instead of wanting *results* right now. Remember that the good stuff takes time. Don't compare the speed of your progress to anyone else's; they are not you. Just do you!

7. Thou shalt . . . keep going when the going gets tough (because it will)

It is best I tell you this now: there will be moments when you can't do it, or you miss a session, or you walk away thinking you didn't try hard enough, or it didn't feel as successful as before. But you turned up and you tried, so draw a line under it and move on. If you give up, you certainly won't get there. Focus on celebrating effort rather than results. I always tell myself to treat each session as a new event; I consider how I am feeling that day and adjust my expectations accordingly. Are you going to be able to train well if you have been up half the night with a screaming baby, or had a few tequilas at the office party the night before? No. So just focus on turning up and making the effort, and celebrate small successes.

When a session feels tough, I focus on 'talking to myself' rather than 'listening to myself'. This is something Nike Global Master Trainer Joslyn Thompson Rule once said to me, and it has stuck. If you just listen, you hear your body complaining and asking to stop because you're tired or it's raining or you have a hangover. If your body and mind are risk-averse, you are never going to make progress (if you are in pain or you feel ill, that's different, so do stop). But when it's my motivation that's looking tragic, I find it is helpful to talk to myself – sternly if necessary – to coach myself through just the next one minute or the next set, to try to give myself that bit of extra fire.

Know that if you are truly pushing your limits to build a stronger, more resilient body and mind there will be times when you fail, and that's okay. We are taught growing up that failure is bad, to worry about what everyone will think if we can't do it. But I actually enjoy failure as it means I have found my limit and I tried – and one day I WILL get there. So many times in life I have avoided doing something for fear of looking stupid and getting it wrong, and I bet you have too. But with weight-lifting you are not going to achieve a personal best every time. Sometimes we have to fail and learn to come back and try it again. Failure doesn't mean the end, it means try again, and again, until you get there. And you will!

It helps to set yourself small and achievable goals, whether that's aiming to complete your planned number of sessions for that week or to increase the load on a lift, or just purely to enjoy your session. Confidence is to be found in your own efforts, so keep turning up, stay the course, do what you enjoy and get s**t done!

If you are new to lifting, you are likely to encounter something called DOMS, or delayed onset muscle soreness. This is when your muscles complain a day or two after you've worked them (also known as collapsing into a chair and not being able to get up!). Sometimes, if you have pushed yourself really hard and you are a beginner, DOMS can hang around for up to three or four days afterwards. It sounds alarming but all it means is that you have overloaded the muscle. You have made it do something it hasn't done before. When I first started Cross-Fit, OMG the soreness was insane. For that first month or two I could hardly move; I was like R2D2 in the shower. But if you keep training, your muscles eventually adapt to the stimulus, as mine did, and you won't hurt as much. DOMS sounds bad but it's actually a sign that you are increasing your fitness. So don't let it put you off.

You can still train, but it probably isn't the greatest idea to kick something when it's down. So give yourself a day or two to recover before going again. Instead, maybe do something low impact like going for a swim or training light on the bike to keep moving and keep up the blood flow to the muscles. Sometimes people think if you are not getting DOMS you haven't worked hard enough, but that's rubbish. You don't need to feel soreness to know you have done a decent workout.

8. Thou shalt . . . swerve the bulls**t

If I have to watch another bum angle shot from yet another terrible workout video . . .

The internet and social media are amazing tools to inspire people and showcase different ways to train, and I'm a massive fan of Instagram as you probably know – it has enabled me to connect and inspire and be inspired by many. However, there are things to bear in mind, mainly that the internet isn't governed in any sense. So everyone and anyone can change their Instagram bio to 'FIT PRO' and we all then assume they should know what they are talking about. So, if I just do this booty band workout five times a week, drink this detox tea or that protein shake, I should look like they do? Err, no. Sadly, life doesn't work like that. Companies pay 'influencers' to peddle their products; it's just another form of advertising but it's masquerading as truth and reality. Surely a well known celebrity with shedloads of followers wouldn't put up an airbrushed, edited photo of themselves, would they? They wouldn't try to sell me something that they don't actually use themselves, would they? I have to say it makes me cross that these people are creating a wholly unrealistic aspiration for so many of us. But we know better than that – we wish them the best and we move on.

Over the years we have been shown images of what 'health' should look like: muscle-ripped men and 'toned' women with visible abs and very little body fat. You see these images all the time on the front cover of fitness magazines. But how real are they? If you have made it to the front cover you will have prepared quite rigorously for the photoshoot (obviously, you would want to look your best). These people are either genetically gifted, and/or have been training really hard potentially for years to get to that point. Then there's the editing: very few pictures make it to the front cover without a fair degree of 'brushing'. Then the headline will say, 'Get Abs in 7 Easy Moves'. Well, no, it doesn't work like that. How do you get a six-pack? Yes, training abs is important, but hundreds of sit-ups alone, with the occasional juice cleanse thrown in, won't do it. It's compound lifts and isolation work that will train your abdominals and then, depending on the individual, your body fat percentage will determine whether those abs are visible or not. We all have abs – some are stronger than others, some are more visible than others. You can have the strongest abs in the world, but if they are covered by a layer of body fat, you won't see them.

Most recently, popping glutes and a small waist has been the trend, so we have seen women everywhere doing squat pulses hoping to get a Kardashian-style bottom. Will it work? To be honest, it's unlikely you will get Khloe K's bum. Don't get me wrong, I have also fallen for these kind of quick-fix solutions when I didn't know what else to try. But they don't work in isolation. What works for one person may not work for another, not to mention the importance of other factors such as diet, sleep, stress levels, recovery and genetics.

Get your information and advice from a fitness professional, and remember that if the results of that 'miracle workout plan' look a bit too good to be true, they probably are. If it looks a bit complicated, or it looks like a marketing pitch, run for the hills (which will probably improve your fitness much better than that 'miracle workout' anyway).

So forget what anyone else is doing. This has to be for you, because you love and value your body enough to look after it. It's a work in progress, but it's also the most important project you will ever work on. Sure, use social media to inspire you, but as soon as it starts to have a detrimental effect, remove yourself from it, as it's not serving you. Be careful who you follow, be sure that they practise what they preach, and that they are open to different methods (that's always a good sign that they understand the fundamental principles of fitness.)

Swerve all the bulls**t methods and quick fixes. It will take the time it takes. All we can do is focus on our plan, enjoy the journey and forget the noise around us.

9. Thou shalt . . . rest and recover

Here we go, full disclosure here. I used to truly feel like if I wasn't making the most of every spare second, training as hard and as often as I possibly could, I was slowing my results down. I constantly felt like I wasn't doing enough; I didn't know how to slow down, to pace myself. But that's where it went wrong for me, and I ended up hurting my lower back, which put me out of training for several weeks. Those weeks felt like a lifetime. But, do you know what? When I was able to return, it felt like my body had really celebrated the rest, and I genuinely think I came back stronger.

It was a good lesson that rest and recovery are absolutely key in the journey to strength. Everyone needs rest days away from training. If you are new to lifting, you certainly don't want to start by doing it seven days a week; it isn't sustainable and you may injure yourself.

I advise scheduling in a 'deload week' every 8–10 weeks for experienced lifters, or every 4–6 weeks if you are a beginner. That's where you bring down the frequency or the weight or intensity to about 60 per cent of your usual plan to allow your body to make a better recovery, as it adapts to all the training stimuli. During that week, keep the body moving and stay active but at a lower intensity. We are in this for the long haul, remember, so let your central nervous system relax a bit. That way, your body gets an extended period of time to recover and bank all your training gains.

A good night's sleep is also incredibly important for your health. In fact, it's just as important as eating healthy and exercising. Unfortunately, modern life has a habit of interfering with our natural sleep patterns. It is thought that people are now sleeping fewer hours than they did fifty years ago, and the quality of that sleep has also declined. None of us is immune here. It is just so, so hard to turn off your phone earlier in the evening and not check what your friend John's ex was doing in Mexico in 2014. The internet is one giant rabbit hole: once you start going down it you burrow deeper and deeper and suddenly you look up and it's 1am. And if you're supposed to be up at 5am that's a sure case of 'see ya later good mood'.

Sleep deprivation can impact your performance and also your motivation to get out and do everything you wanted. If I haven't had seven or eight hours sleep I know I won't be as good as I was the day before. If I've been out and had a few drinks and crashed into bed at 1am, I can't expect my body to function well: it's like trying to drive a car with no petrol in it.

It is true that the real gains of training occur during the recovery. It's when you are asleep that your body recovers from the stresses you have put it through during your workout; it is busy repairing all those muscle fibres so they can come back bigger and stronger. If you are trying to lose weight as well, good-quality sleep is absolutely critical. Studies show that sleep-deprived people have a bigger appetite and tend to eat more calories, especially from poor-quality carbs (I've *so* been there). Scientists think this is because sleep deprivation disrupts the hormones that govern our appetite, telling us to stop eating when we are full.[13]

When it comes to how much sleep you need, everyone is different. But don't kid yourself that you are one of those people who can survive on just a few hours. The number of people who can thrive on tiny amounts of sleep is absolutely minuscule. Most people need at least seven hours, and eight is even better. So don't spend all night looking at your phone; try to put it aside at least an hour before bedtime and get into bed early enough to give you that magic shut-eye.

10. Thou shalt . . . respect the process

So, this is where I tell you that there is no cheating the process. Patience has to be your best friend. There may be days when you see great results, others when you feel you may have hit a plateau. Be mindful of these feelings, observe them, reassess your plan, check your adherence to the plan and re-evaluate. It takes time to get strong, so be kind to yourself and don't expect instant results. You are training for life, don't forget, not to look better in a photo next Saturday night.

If you are a beginner and you stick to your plan of strength training two or three times a week, while also upping your general activity levels and eating well, you will probably see changes to your body in four to six weeks – perhaps even a bit earlier (but definitely not in seven days). We all adapt at different rates, so do all of the above, be consistent, make it a part of your lifestyle and enjoy the journey.

It's important to know that one 'bad' day of food, or a missed training session doesn't define you. So just because you had a night out then ate a packet of biscuits you found in a drawer at work the next day, it doesn't wreck all the positive gains you have made so far, so don't let it! Draw a line under it, move on and get back to the plan. That happened to me very recently while I was halfway through a 42-day calorie deficit to help my training for the marathon. Over three days of socializing one weekend I ate maybe 1,000 calories more than I should have done according to my plan – mainly in alcohol and chocolate, if I'm honest. I felt a bit annoyed about it at first, but I also had to remember that in the days before that I probably built up a deficit of 2,000 calories. So over the whole week, I was still on the right side of the energy-in energy-out equation for fat loss, just not as much as I could have been. But no one is perfect and no one can eat broccoli every day. You can't always sacrifice everything, especially when you have social occasions on the calendar. You are the result of the decisions you make consistently, not the thing you did that one time you had a Mars bar or a crisp sandwich. It's about allowing yourself some leeway, forgiving yourself and moving on with new vitality and a bit of a spring in your step.

'LIFT, SLEEP, EAT WELL, HAVE FUN, STRESS LESS AND THE RESULTS WILL COME.'

4· GETTING STARTED

By now you are hopefully raring to go lift something, but better put your nan back down on the sofa (carefully) while I give you a little bit of information on how to do it safely, as well as how to build up an effective training routine that will help you achieve your goals. Which may or may not include lifting your nan.

Rushing in head first (or legs first) is not a good idea. Lifting has to be done correctly or you may injure yourself. At the very least, if you are not executing the moves properly, you won't get the full benefits from your training.

If you are an absolute beginner, you can start training on your own, at home, using some basic weights, and I will tell you more about how to do that later on. But I would really recommend you start by seeking guidance from a professional who can assess your fitness and advise you how to structure your training and avoid excess load and injury.

Here are your best options:

- Go to a beginner's strength circuit class. I am a huge advocate of these as, if they are delivered properly, the instructor will be able to give you some guidance on form and technique. They may also use some of the gym equipment that you might feel too intimidated to try on your own. The good thing about a class is that you're in a group and everyone is too busy focusing on their own form to notice what you are doing. No hiding at the back, though.

- See a personal trainer. Believe me, they are not at all scary or intimidating. Everyone was new to this once, including them. A good personal trainer will assess you and guide you through a do-able plan depending on your goals – whether that's to get fitter, to get stronger or to lose fat (or all three). They will show you how to use the machines at the gym, and how to use free weights like dumbbells and kettlebells effectively. Check out free trial offers at your local gym, or you could get together with a friend to share the cost. I would say that consulting a personal trainer is especially important if you have any injuries or physical limitations.

- Go DIY, but check your form on the internet, following professional sources (like me). Yes, you can make this journey on your own, but you need to be really careful to make sure you are lifting correctly. In the next chapter I have listed the twenty key moves that you are likely to see in my beginner's lifting plan. If you are flying solo, I want you to promise me that you will check how the move should be executed . . . I will ensure these are available for you, so you can watch me do them first online. When you try out the exercises, a good idea is to set up your phone so you can video your session and look at your form. Everyone will naturally move a little differently but the principles will be the same. Be your own coach!

Before you start, make sure you are wearing clothing and shoes fit for purpose. I know this might sound obvious, and this isn't always about splashing out on expensive, technologically advanced sportswear, but you need to wear something comfortable and supportive. Most importantly, wear supportive shoes. I own over one hundred pairs of training shoes, and although I completely agree that this is a tad excessive, I have different shoes for different types of physical work, such as running shoes with a slight turn up in the toe to help with forward momentum and shoes specifically for lifting, which need to provide flat and secure contact with the floor.

There are lots of different types of resistance training. If you are a beginner, you won't need to know about all of these just yet, but I think it's important to understand the basics before you get going. Here are some that I have used:

- **Body weight** This is where you execute a move – say a squat or a plank – with only your body weight for resistance. This is where it's best to start as a beginner before adding in any weights.

- **Machine-based resistance** Yep, that means all those scary-looking machines at the gym. Except that they're not that scary once you've been shown how to use them properly.

- **Free weights** You are doing similar work to what you do on the machines, but using weights you hold in your hands. At the beginner stage, that would mainly be dumbbells and a kettlebell – and you can use these at home too.

- **Weightlifting** This is generally barbell work – that's the classic long weightlifting bar where you add weights at each end. This is for more advanced lifters who have already had some experience in the three types of training above. These lifts generally involve more complex or compound movements.

- **Plyometrics** This is a very intense form of training, where your muscles are exerting maximal force in a very short space of time – think jump squats or jumping lunges. It brings explosiveness and speed to a move in order to increase power.

Your body contains hundreds of muscles (at least 650, and up to 840 depending on how you count them). So how do you know which ones to work? You may be grateful to hear that I am not proposing 840 different exercises. What we tend to concentrate on are the big groups of muscles that we use every day just living our lives. Think about what muscles you're using when you carry heavy shopping bags, or quickly move out of the way of a closing train door, pull something off a high shelf or chase your child when they have decided to leg it out of the playground. All of these kinds of moves come under the heading of functional fitness – that's fitness with a real-life everyday purpose, where your muscles are working together in a stable and strong movement pattern.

So, for example, imagine picking up a heavy bag from the floor. As you bend from the hips you use some of your body's most powerful muscles, like the gluteal muscles in your bum, core and lower back. That hinging movement is pretty much what you are doing when you deadlift, which is one of the key moves in lifting. In fact, it has been called the king (or queen!) of lifts because it uses so many of your major muscle groups.

To take another example, say you want to grab something from the bottom drawer or shelf of your fridge. You would naturally squat down and up again, which uses your glutes, hamstrings and core muscles. Squatting is such a natural human movement that small children can often sit completely comfortably in that position for ages, yet as adults we find it far harder because our glutes are out of practice from inactivity or sitting in chairs for too long. A squat is another key move in strength training, and one that will benefit you hugely in real life.

Some questions (and answers) for the beginner

By now, you probably have lots of questions about how to get started with weights, and what a typical workout might look like. So here we go:

Should I be training every day?

No! As a beginner or intermediate lifter, please don't feel the pressure to join team #nodaysoff because you really do need to have adequate rest and recovery days for your body to repair itself.

I would say that as a beginner, you should aim for one hour of strength training a week in either two sessions of 30 minutes or three sessions of 20 minutes. The advantage of doing two 30-minute sessions is that you get two clear days off between each session to maximize your recovery time. That doesn't mean you should lie on your sofa on those two days, though. It's good to mix your strength training with cardiovascular conditioning. Depending on your fitness, that could be an aerobics class, a run or HIIT (high-intensity interval training). It could just be a brisk 30-minute walk in your lunch break. All activity counts.

As you progress with your strength training, you could increase your sessions to three or four a week as you feel appropriate. No rush.

What exercises are best, and how many should I do?

The most effective ones are going to be the ones that work multiple muscle groups, rather than isolating individual muscles. These are called compound movements, and include exercises like the squat, the press-up, the deadlift and the lunge. You will find out more about these exercises in the next chapter.

Ideally, you want to do 10–12 of your chosen exercise (we call that 10–12 reps) then have a rest, then do that 'set' of 10–12 reps two or three more times. Depending on your starting fitness you may not be able to complete that to begin with, but it's a good target to have.

Those last two or three reps should be a struggle, but you should still be maintaining correct form. If you find it impossible to do the exercise properly because your muscles are too tired, then it's safer to stop and lower your target for that day. It's not a race, and slow and steady progress is key.

In a beginner's workout, you might get through six or seven different exercises in a 20- or 30-minute session, but that really depends on your fitness and how you are feeling that day. Not every day is going to be an amazing training day.

How heavy should my weights be?

To start with, I suggest not using weights at all. Sound weird? Let me explain. If you are just using your body weight, you will be able to focus on your technique and perfect the movement without worrying about having to lift something at the same time. As you know by now, the way you lift (your 'form') is crucial. Film yourself doing the moves and compare them with my Technique School in the next chapter.

When it comes to strength training it's a case of quality over quantity: start with the basics, master the foundational movement patterns in the next chapter and once you feel confident, you can start to work with resistance.

When you progress to weights, broadly speaking you need to pick a weight that challenges you, but doesn't break you. If you are a complete beginner, then a 3kg dumbbell might be a good place to start. It's not about how heavy that weight is, but how much effort it requires from you to lift it. Ideally, you want to be able to complete your chosen number of reps, and if by that last rep it feels challenging, that's a good thing, as long as you are still lifting it correctly in a controlled movement. Find a weight with which you can complete the given reps with good form and think about always trying to finish with one or two reps left in the tank. Remember to write down the weights you used and how many reps and sets you completed and refer back to them when you repeat the session.

What equipment should I buy?

The world really is your gym, now that you can buy good-quality weights for £10–20 in high-street shops like Argos and sports shops, or from online retailers such as Amazon or Europe's largest strength and conditioning equipment manufacturer Bulldog Gear. But don't go out just yet and fill your garage with expensive machines you've seen on QVC.

You actually don't need much equipment for an effective beginner's strength training workout. If you are doing your strength training at home I would advise buying a pair of basic dumbbells (those coloured Neoprene ones you see in the shops are absolutely fine). They come in weights from 1kg to about 10kg. To find the weight that's right for you, I suggest going into the shop and trying them out. Perhaps go for the 3kg and press it above your head ten times. Then ask yourself how hard that was on a scale of 1 to 10. If it was a 7, then that's probably about right for you, but a score much lower than that and you should try a heavier weight. I wouldn't even bother trying the 1kg or 2kg weights. When you think that the average woman's handbag weighs 2.4kg, you have to wonder what's the point of trying to strength train with something lighter than the bag you carry around all day!

Once you get going with your strength training, I would also advise buying a kettlebell. This is a solid ball-shaped weight with a handle, and it is great for increasing the intensity of moves such as squats and deadlifts. Again, go to a shop and try one out before you choose your weight; 8kg can be a good one to start with.

How do I know when to increase the weight?

There should be absolutely no rush to increase the weight. Your first priority should always be to master the technique and the range of motion. For example, in a squat you should aim to hit good depth before you start to bring in additional resistance. So take it slow, and remember that there are lots of other ways you can increase intensity without increasing the weight.

Here are some ways to increase intensity:

- More reps/sets with the same weight

- Better range of motion, form and technique with the same weight

- More 'time under tension' with the same weight. Essentially that means instead of purely lifting it and putting it back down again, we can slow down either the lifting part of the movement (the concentric) or the lowering part (the eccentric). We call this 'adding a tempo'. For example, in a normal set of 10–12 reps of an exercise, the muscle could be under tension for a total of 25–30 seconds. If we were to add a tempo, a '3-second eccentric' would increase the muscle time under tension by another 10–15 seconds, making the muscle work relatively harder, without increasing the weight

- Less rest time with the same weight

- More speed/control with the same weight

- And then, finally, you could increase the weight

Don't get hung up on the idea that increasing the weight is the most important goal. It is important, but it is not the only way to progress.

When you first start your training, you will notice that your rate of improvement is rapid, but as you get stronger the gains will be slower and harder to attain. That's what people mean when they talk about a training plateau, where you seem to be getting more comfortable with your plan. But if you stay here for too long, you are not giving your muscles the necessary stimulus to adapt and grow. 'Progressive overload' is the key here. What do I mean by that? In essence it means gradually increasing the demands you make of your muscles. For example, if you were to go to the gym and do exactly the same full-body workout with exactly the same weights, reps and sets for years and years, you might not see any changes to your body because you are no longer challenging your muscles to work harder; you are just maintaining a level. Those muscles have got pretty comfortable doing their thing! They need an increase in the stimulus to help them grow and you will only progress by making changes to your overall training volume:

more reps, more sets, more weights, less rest. In other words, progressively overloading it.

As a guide, you are looking for something between 5 and 8 per cent added to the resistance per week. Always remember there are so many factors that may affect your performance, so just see where you are at that particular session, and make decisions about weights appropriately. Don't let your ego make you feel like you need to be making big progress fast.

How can I develop my strength?

Once you have mastered the basics and introduced some weights into your training, it's up to you how you progress. It all depends on what your goals are: are you looking to be fitter and more defined, or have you got the strength bug and want to take your training up a notch? Here are some basic goals and ways to achieve them:

- To get fitter and look toned, you will probably want to stick with a relatively high number of reps with lighter weights. That would generally be 8–12 reps per set, and three or four sets of relatively basic movement patterns. Rest is purposefully quite minimal, perhaps 60 seconds between sets.

- To build muscle (called hypertrophy) you will still be working in the 8–12 rep range. You may use barbells, free weights or machines.

- To maximize strength, you will generally work with heavier weights but because it's hugely taxing on the body you will typically do far fewer reps, perhaps 3–5 maximum. You will also need to add in 3–5 minutes of rest between sets to allow your body to recover.

'THE BEST ADVICE I CAN GIVE IS TO LISTEN TO YOUR BODY.'

Should I warm up?

Yes, this is absolutely essential because it prepares your body for the moves it is about to do, and excites your nervous system for what lies ahead. A warm-up, by the way, isn't touch your toes, circle your knees, do ten star jumps and slap yourself in the face . . . This is one of my greatest peeves as a coach, not preparing the body sufficiently. In its broadest sense, warming up is mobilizing, activating and preparing the muscles for the exercises you are about to do and telling your body it is about to work.

A common mistake among lifters is that they don't put enough focus on the warm-up and specific movement preparation. You don't want to start lifting weights after just doing a brisk jog on the treadmill – sure it may fire you up mentally and raise your heart rate slightly, but that's not very specific is it? Really think about what movements you are about to perform and prepare your body for them. If you are going to squat heavy in your session, then there is no better way to prepare for that than practising that movement in your warm-up, just at a lower intensity.

So ensure your warm-up doesn't just consist of a couple of planks and some arm and leg shakes. Use mobility drills and dynamic stretching to open up and switch on particular areas before you start to move with more intensity. This will help to prevent injury and allow your body to move to a greater potential.

After your training, it is also good practice to cool down, especially if you are a beginner. If you have elevated your heart rate, some stretching work afterwards will give you time to return to your normal state and give your body the chance to reset. Active stretching generally involves moving a limb at a joint through its full range of motion to the end ranges and then repeating. It could also reduce the build-up of lactic acid in your muscles, which is what gives you that burning feeling deep into a workout and can lead to cramping and stiffness. Stretch the muscles you have worked, but also maybe the ones you haven't, holding each position for at least 10 seconds. Give yourself time to focus on your breath and take a few moments to reflect on the work you have done and what you have achieved in your session.

How tired should I feel?

If you are a beginner and you have managed three sets of say 10 reps of an exercise, then you should be feeling pretty knackered! In the fitness world we use a scale called RPE (rate of perceived exertion), which describes your effort level from 1 to 10, with 10 being completely out of breath or challenging close to the point of failure. When I am doing HIIT training, I would describe my RPE as a 9 or a 10 because in HIIT you are working at high intensity with a short recovery time. On a big lifting session, on my last set, for those last reps you will see my face completely screwed up, hating every second of it, because that burn is so challenging.

With strength training you should feel a slightly different level of RPE, depending on the number of sets and reps. It should feel a little more manageable because it is largely short anaerobic work. That means it involves short bursts of intense force rather than the longer periods of steadier exercise you get in aerobic activities like running. But as the volume of the weights increases, you will definitely feel the burn! When you are a beginner, I would advise leaving two full days between sessions.

During a strength training session, how long you rest for in between sets will vary hugely depending on your level, and how you are training based on your goal. If you are lifting lighter weights with higher reps, you might only have 60 seconds between each set. But if you are a well-trained individual and have progressed to heavier weights at lower reps, for maximal strength gains, you will need a longer rest time in between sets, somewhere between 1–3 minutes, to enable you to recover enough to lift again at a higher percentage of your maximum capability. But if you're a beginner, you don't need to worry about this for now.

How do I stop myself getting injured?

Moving safely should always be your priority over intensity, and it is important to engage and brace your core, to stabilize the spine to protect us from injury, completing the full range of motion (as much as your mobility allows) throughout all lifts. It's also good to remember that it's cool being mobile, but we need to be strong in these positions too. I always say that if it doesn't feel right, it probably isn't, so don't force it and push it further than you are comfortable with. Either reduce the weight, amend the reps or just come back to that movement another time.

With weightlifting there can be a tendency to feel like you are only progressing if you are lifting more, but progress isn't always steady and linear. There will be times where you can't increase the intensity because you were out late last night or don't feel great. If I achieved a personal best every week I have been training, I would be at the Olympics by now! So listen to your body and be prepared to adapt your plan accordingly. Know the difference between effort and ability that day.

Overtraining is a real thing, and you need to be aware of it. I want you to try to be aware of the intensity you are working at and remember that exercise is a stress to the body. So for example, it's not a good idea to do a HIIT workout three or four days in a row, because you'll be working at 90 per cent of your maximum heart rate, and it takes some time for your body to recover. With strength training you can work at different intensities across the week: some days you may go relatively 'heavy' whereas other days may be more volume-based (lighter weights with more reps). Believe me, I was that person who overtrained. I had found this thing that made me so happy and had given me this new lease of life so I wanted to do it all the time, but my body couldn't keep up; I was overtraining and under-recovering. It's like the bus in the film *Speed*: it's going so fast you know it's not going to end well, but you don't seem to be able to stop it. So, speaking from experience as someone who has crashed and burned, stick to the plan and don't feel the need to do more.

As you know, one of the ways I advise avoiding overtraining is by scheduling in a 'deload week' (see page 79). This is where you bring down the volume, the frequency, or the weight/intensity to about 60 per cent of your usual plan. That allows the body to make a better recovery, and adapt to all the training stimuli you're giving it. Keep the body moving and stay active during your deload week, just at a lower intensity.

What happens if I can't lift a weight?

The best advice I can give is to listen to your body. If you are struggling it may be that you have chosen a weight that's too heavy for you right now. If you selected a pair of dumbbells for 10–12 reps of a shoulder press and you only completed six before feeling that your arms were dropping off, that was probably too heavy. However, if you could have done 112, maybe they were too light. You need to find a weight that feels challenging for you for the specific workout format.

If one day the same weight feels much heavier than it did before, it could be a sign that your muscles have not yet repaired from the previous session. Or maybe you haven't had a decent night's sleep, or your stress levels are high or you haven't eaten well. This happens to everyone, no matter how well trained they are. Sometimes I pick something up that should be manageable and I just have to say to myself, wow, this is not the one for today. I reduce my expectation of myself and just go with what feels right and challenging. If it doesn't feel right or you feel pain in any lifts, don't push it, and always consult a professional who can assess you.

My muscles are sore three days afterwards: is this normal?

Absolutely, yes! This is called DOMS (delayed onset muscle soreness) and it's very common in beginners. If you can hardly bend down to put your shoes on or get in the car without lifting your legs in, then you have a case of DOMS. Even more experienced lifters get DOMS when they are trying something new.

DOMS happens because when you use a muscle in a way you haven't done before, you are causing little micro tears in that muscle. That sounds frightening, but it's actually a positive thing because when the muscle repairs, it comes back firmer and stronger. It's a sign your fitness is progressing. But during the repair process, it can be pretty sore. DOMS usually strikes 24 hours after your session and if you are lucky, you might get away with having it for 24 hours. But if you have worked really intensively in a new movement pattern for you, you might still be feeling sore three or four days afterwards. However, I do want to stress that you don't need to get DOMS to prove you have worked hard; you can do a great workout without it.

There is no magic treatment for getting rid of DOMS, but make sure you stay hydrated and eat plenty of protein. Rugby players often jump in an ice bath, which might be a bit extreme for most of us, but if you want to give it a go, be my guest! Gentle exercise like walking helps too, because it keeps the blood flowing to your muscles. You can still train if you are sore, but I'd take the intensity down and give your body a rest for a couple of days. Concentrate on low-impact exercise like swimming instead. The day after I did the London Marathon in 2013, I genuinely couldn't sit down or stand up, I just 'fell' everywhere. My mum really enjoyed taking me to a spa that day; she just plopped me into the jacuzzi and we stayed there for hours.

Do I need to be taking a protein powder?

First of all, remember that a protein powder is a supplement, and in my mind, this is just what it is: something that is *additional* to your nutrition. So yes, you absolutely can if you find it difficult to get sufficient protein in your current diet. But I would always suggest you aim to get as much of it as possible from real food sources before looking at supplements.

Protein is an important component of your diet when you are strength training because it is needed for building and repairing muscles and other tissues. How much you eat a day depends on your goals: someone training for a Strongwoman competition is going to need more than a beginner lifter doing strength training twice a week. We looked at how much you might need in Chapter 3 (see page 70), but it could be anything from 50g a day (the UK's daily recommended amount) to 100+g a day. Given that an average 150g chicken breast contains about 48g of protein, you can see it should be pretty straightforward to build enough into your diet if you're eating well, even as a vegetarian. Good sources of protein are: meat, fish, cheese, tofu, beans, lentils, yoghurt/dairy, nuts and seeds.

What exercise should I be doing alongside my strength training?

To be the best version of you as an everyday athlete, I don't believe you should be doing solely strength training, not even those whose goal is gaining some serious strength. Cardio exercise is a vital part of your overall exercise 'diet'. The UK Government recommends a minimum of two and a half hours of moderate-intensity aerobic exercise per week – the kind of exercise that makes you a little bit gassed but you can still just about talk. That could be running, cycling, brisk walking or aerobics classes – whatever you love doing. I am not joking when I say you have to find something you are passionate about, because you won't be able to keep doing the thing you hate. Do it with a pal for a bit of social accountability. Whatever lights you fire, DO THAT.

Your strength training is on top of these 150 minutes. If you are a beginner and you do two sessions a week, then do your cardio-based exercise on the other days rather than on the same day if you can. Once you get more experienced, and if you are a bit tight for time, you could run the sessions together, but always do your strength training first while you have full energy levels, and do your cardio work afterwards with whatever energy you have left.

Whichever cardio exercise you choose, it's important to maximize your general activity levels, too. It all counts when it comes to burning fat and establishing a healthy, non-sedentary lifestyle. The fitness industry is never short of fancy terminology, so let me introduce you to LISS and NEAT. LISS (low-intensity steady state) is gentle exercise like walking or cycling that's done at a relaxed pace over a continuous period. NEAT (non-exercise activity thermogenesis) is all the energy you use when you're not eating, sleeping or taking 'Exercise' with a capital E. It's basically a posh way of saying walk instead of taking the bus, or get up every hour at work to walk to the photocopier. Ideally, you want to be maximizing both LISS and NEAT in your life. It doesn't need to be too complicated; exercise is movement, across different intensities.

When it comes to my own life, I do a mix of all these things. Because of my work, I'm naturally very active and have quite a high step count in my day (over 20,000 steps marching around a gym!) so that means plenty of LISS and NEAT. Cardio-wise, I find HIIT works for me alongside my strength training. It is incredibly intense and works my cardiovascular system to the extreme, and because it doesn't take long it's also time-efficient. I weirdly enjoy diving into the pain cave of this type of cardio work. I love a challenge and I am not afraid of hard work – it feels horrendous at the time but it's a mind game. Your body can do it; it's just about how far you can push yourself before your mind takes over. But there are no rules; find the exercise you love because that's the one you will stick at in the long term.

What if I fall off the wagon?

It happens to everyone at some point. Really. Even those Instagram FIT PROS who seem to live in the gym are going to have times when they just can't do it. Maybe they're not even doing it! (Honestly, don't believe half of what you see on Instagram because I have witnessed it: filming a couple of reps, and then posting that they had done the whole thing in whatever time.) So do not compare yourselves to strangers on the internet; instead focus on your own achievement.

The road is not clear or straight. We are all individuals with complicated lives, and there will be many things that can impact your training and your motivation every single day: a bad day at work, an argument with your other half – it all has an impact. We just have to prioritize giving ourselves this time no matter what. In committing to getting stronger and fitter, you are developing good habits and making daily sensible choices. So if you miss your training one day, well, fine. No big deal, make it up another time. We are creating positive habits, not punishing ourselves for our high expectations.

We mustn't kill ourselves to hit the goal, we must do what makes us happy. One 'bad' day of food, or one missed training session doesn't define you; it's what you do frequently that counts. We are the result of what we consistently do.

Strength training: our journeys

Using my own experiences, my life's purpose is now to share my journey with as many people as possible, connecting with people who find strength in losing themselves in a session, and showing how strength training has the potential to change their lives for the better. Don't get me wrong; it isn't going to solve all your problems, but I know I am so much more optimistic and collected in tough situations now and much more accepting of myself. So, I have the pleasure of sharing these stories with you. Meet some more of Team LIFTED – they can tell you first-hand what it's like to start on a lifting and fitness journey. I hope you find their stories – and their honesty – inspiring.

Emma Dart, 38, Rotherham

To me, strength means pushing my body to see what it can do, and understanding that building a strong body and mind now will help me to stay physically and mentally fitter in older age.

'ONE "BAD" DAY
OF FOOD, OR ONE
MISSED TRAINING
SESSION DOESN'T
DEFINE YOU;
IT'S WHAT YOU
DO FREQUENTLY
THAT COUNTS. WE
ARE THE RESULT
OF WHAT WE
CONSISTENTLY DO.'

About four years ago I reached a plateau with cardio-based weight loss. At that time my step-daughter started to stay overnight with us every week; I wanted to be stronger to be able to help care for her – she's 13 now and has quadriplegic cerebral palsy and can't walk so needs to be lifted. A local personal trainer was re-establishing his business after some time off with ill health and offered me six months of free strength training in return for documenting my journey for his marketing campaign. It was an offer I couldn't refuse and I have never looked back.

I gained a sense of achievement as well as a way to relieve stress. I find it gives me a space to zone everything out and focus on me for 30/45/60 minutes without the worry of work, washing, ironing and everyday life. I love the rush when you hit a new PB (personal best). Training makes me stronger in body and mind and I love how my body has changed as a result of lifting.

My advice to any first-timers would be to just start! Make sure you find someone to train you that you're comfortable with, know your initial goal (it WILL change as you progress) and just take that first step! I wish I'd found lifting sooner, instead of wasting years yo-yoing with cardio just to drop a dress size for a holiday or Christmas party.

Katherine, 28, Essex

A gym opened up in an old warehouse at the end of my road. I drove past it every day for about nine months, and I always saw people coming out looking hot and sweaty but so happy. I had only ever had horrible experiences at gyms but something about this one felt different. I was struggling with my weight, fitness and general self-esteem and I decided just to pluck up the courage and go in. I started working with an epic personal trainer and now I can't imagine my life without weightlifting.

Since I started training I have learned so much about my body: how to look after it, how to nourish it, as well as looking after myself mentally. I have made some incredible lifelong friends, some of whom I would never have crossed paths with had I not joined that gym. Training has given me the confidence to take part in weightlifting competitions, run half-marathons, complete Tough Mudders – all things I have always wanted to try but never dared to before. Feeling strong makes me feel like I can conquer the world. Once you've lifted more than your body weight, you can do anything, right?

My advice would be to find a gym you love and if you don't find one straight away, keep looking. Experiment with different types of training. There are so many options out there that there will definitely be something for you. If it's weightlifting you're interested in, just pick up a weight, write everything down, monitor and track your progress, and you'll see the gains arrive in no time.

Ella, 25, London

The journey to fit isn't always easy. I recently completed a ten-week fitness and strength training challenge, and there were times when my motivation really sagged. I think the toughest thing was waking up and travelling for an hour at 6am to make a class, especially as it got colder. That made me start to miss classes and try to move my schedule around. I found myself having to balance everything and say no to outings and working late as I needed to reserve my energy for training. Waking up and motivating myself became more and more difficult at the halfway point. Although I could see slight changes in my body and my face, I was feeling heavy, tired and very sore!

The turning point was definitely at week six when someone at work said, 'Wow you look skinny!' I know this was a great exaggeration but I then noticed my once-tight Topshop jeans were sagging at the waist and constantly falling down, and my favourite coat started to make me look like an elf (due to the increased room around the arms and stomach area) – even my shoes were loose. This was when I believe I went into 'beast' mode and started going extra hard, even adding sessions on the weekend at another gym!

The ten-week challenge definitely changed my life. The best thing about the whole experience has been learning what my body can actually do and pushing myself to a level of fitness I could only ever dream of before. I now know that physically and mentally I am more than capable of achieving any fitness goal I set my mind to, and I have stopped telling myself 'no' before I have even tried to achieve anything. I am determined to keep going and I hope this is the start of major fitness changes that will last my whole life.

Zoe Rogers, 30, London

I was a severely overweight child and teenager and only really started understanding fitness about three years ago. I feel that lifting and weight training has given me this inner strength and confidence that I'm not sure I would have if I didn't do it. Strength means a lot more to me now: it doesn't just apply to our physical attributes and how much weight we can shift. To me, strength starts at the very top – it's all in our head. We can overcome physical challenges if we have the mental strength to get us there. If we can't battle those pesky demons that are telling us 'no', we'll never get anywhere.

Lifting gave me results, both physically and mentally. I was realizing that I could actually do something and feel good about it – and it was working. It helped build my confidence and give me that drive to work harder and push myself to discover that I was stronger than I gave myself credit for.

For people new to lifting I would encourage them to be as fearless as possible – don't be scared. Your body is amazing and can do pretty much anything you want it to. Lifting will not make you bulky (ladies!), it will make you stronger in so many ways. And never feel intimidated by others. We are all our own person; some people are built better for different things or may have simply been doing it longer than you and had more practice. Take a friend with you, meet new people, make new friends and share the experience of lifting with others – it's a great community. My final word is this: have you ever heard anyone say they like a flat ass? No, of course you haven't. Get lifting.

Helen Cooke, 36, Nottingham

Strength to me means the knowledge that I can lift 'something' without having to think about it – like popping a suitcase up in the luggage rack on a train – real-life, functional, transferable skills. But it's also the feeling of standing up after a heavy squat, or pushing the last inches of a split jerk overhead and letting out a little (okay, big!) growl to help.

By lifting I gained a real sense of achievement and all of a sudden with that came a change in mindset. The realization that actually it doesn't matter what you look like because – look what your body can do! – that's amazing.

My advice to first timers would be to join a club or gym that offers lifting classes. You'll get some structure to your training and hopefully the right support to work on technique and the fundamentals before you move on to the fun stuff of shifting some really heavy iron!

Jay Ann Gardiner, 27, Kent

Strong to me means being strong enough physically to lift the weight, and strong enough mentally to go back the next day and try again.

I have done barbell-based classes on and off for years, but I could feel my form was lacking and I wasn't getting much out of them any more. I contacted a female personal trainer that I felt comfortable with and asked for sessions to teach me correct form and push me beyond my comfort zone. Now I happily train with her, on my own as well as going to functional fitness classes at my local gym and I LOVE IT!

I find it really fun to challenge myself each week, learn a new lift or increase my weight. I have really struggled to find a way of dealing with stress and anxiety, and the endorphins after a great session stick around for days. Lifting really has contributed to how my mental health has improved in the last year. It's an hour to myself where I don't have to worry about anything apart from beating myself.

Katy Moran, 28, London

What does it mean to be strong? When I was a child I imagined men pulling trucks or lifting atlas stones. It is funny to me that it wasn't until I started lifting heavy things myself that I realized strength is about so much more than what you can lift; it is about what you gain when you do. Tenacity, grit, determination, self-appreciation, inner calm and knowing what your body is truly capable of achieving. These are the things that make you strong and I know I found them in myself when I started strength training. It's never too late to get involved in sport and fitness, and there's no limit to your potential. But you'll have to start to see how far you can go.

A lifting glossary

The fitness world can seem intimidating some-times because there is so much technical language, fancy terminology and crazy new acronyms. You don't really need to know that much to get started with lifting, but let me try to demystify some terms a bit for you.

Abs Abbreviation of abdominal muscles, your tummy muscles.

Accessory movement A movement separate from the main lifts, but one that works to complement and strengthen those main lifts. For example, uni-lateral work on a single leg deadlift will improve your overall deadlift. These are mainly used by experienced lifters.

Barbell A long metal weightlifting bar to which you add weights at each end.

Compound lift A movement which uses multiple muscle groups at the same time, such as a squat or a deadlift. These give you the best bang for your buck, strength-wise.

Concentric lift This is the lifting phase of the movement, where your muscle shortens (con-tracts) to generate enough force to lift the weight.

→

Dumbbell A weight that fits into one hand; they are generally used in pairs.

Eccentric lift This is the lowering phase of the lift, where your muscle elongates in response to the force of the weight.

Glutes The gluteal muscles in your bottom, which include the gluteus maximus (your body's largest muscle), the gluteus medius and the gluteus minimus.

Hamstrings The group of three muscles that runs down the back of your thighs.

HIIT High-intensity interval training, or repeated bursts of quick, very high-intensity cardiovascular exercise with rests in between. It can be very effective for improving aerobic fitness and burning calories.

Hypertrophy Muscle hypertrophy means muscle growth. It happens when the size of your muscle cells increase as a result of strength training.

Isolation exercise A movement that works just one muscle group at a time. These are mainly used by bodybuilders to maximize muscle and strength. Compound lifts are more useful for beginners.

Kettlebell Solid, ball-shaped weight with a wide handle across the top.

$\rightarrow$

LISS Low-intensity steady state. This is gentle exercise like walking that's done at a relaxed pace over a continuous period.

Lats Abbreviation of latissimus dorsi, the flat muscles on each side of your mid-back, which are the largest in your upper body.

Muscle fibres These are what make up your muscles. There are two types: fast-twitch muscle fibres, which contract quickly so are good for rapid movements, and slow-twitch muscle fibres, which contract slowly and are good for endurance activities.

NEAT Non-exercise activity thermogenesis. The energy you use when you are not eating, sleeping or doing sport or exercise. An example might be walking up the stairs.

Obliques The external oblique muscles at each side of your abdominals.

PB Personal best; your record for that lift.

Progressive overload Gradually increasing the demands you make of your muscles by giving them increased stimulus to grow.

Quads Abbreviation of quadriceps femoris, the group of four muscles at the front of your thighs.

→

Rep Abbreviation of repetition. Reps are how many repetitions you do of one exercise.

Rhomboids The diamond-shaped muscles on each side of your upper back. They pull the shoulder blades together.

Set A group of reps (repetitions) of an exercise with a rest in between. If you are aiming for three sets of 10 reps, that's 30 reps in total.

Super-set Sets of exercises performed directly after each other to maximize intensity. This is essentially what circuit training is.

Tempo Building in extra time to a lift to increase the time the muscle is under tension. We call it 'adding a tempo'. This is mainly used by experienced lifters.

Traps Abbreviation of trapezoid muscles, the long, flat, triangular-shaped muscles in your upper back.

Unilateral Exercise that works one leg/arm/side of the body not both.

Volume Your training volume means how much work you are getting through: how heavy your weights are, how many reps you are doing and how many sets. It is expressed in this formula: volume = sets x reps x load.

5· TECHNIQUE SCHOOL – A GUIDE TO THE KEY MOVEMENTS TO BUILD STRENGTH

In this chapter I take you through some of the key movement patterns you will see in the world of lifting. They will make you stronger, give you definition and tone, and help your mobility.

It's really important to focus on executing the exercises properly, not only to make sure you don't injure yourself, but also to maximize the full range of motion in each move. Better to do one perfect squat than any number of half-squats, or just-plain-bad squats.

- If any of the moves mention using weights, leave them out at first, and start by using just your body weight. That way you can map and perfect the movement without any distractions.

- Spend time working on perfecting the move slowly before starting your reps.

- Video yourself doing the exercise and compare the footage with the diagrams in this chapter. Are your hips/knees/back/shoulders where they should be?

- Don't forget: everyone's skeletal make-up is different. Appreciate that if you have longer femurs (thigh bones) then your squat may be a little different to those with shorter femurs.

- Always, always, always focus on your form. If you have set yourself 10 reps but at rep 7 you are so tired it's pulling you out of form, rest, reset, reassess and start again.

- Make sure your weight isn't so heavy that it's pulling you out of form by rep 7 – or so light that you could do 100 reps without stopping . . .

- Warm up the movement before you start your workout.

The following are my top moves to master, including information on how, what and why they work.

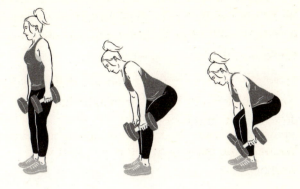

Deadlift

What is it?

This is a compound lift, meaning it uses multiple muscle groups so it's highly effective and efficient. No wonder it is sometimes called the king (or queen!) of all lifts. In simple terms, it is a hip hinge. Think about what you do when you pick something off the floor: hinge at the hips, push your bum back, grab the keys, push the floor away, squeeze your bum, then come back up to full extension, standing up.

How to do it

1. Hold the weights (a dumbbell or kettlebell in each hand) and stand with feet shoulder-width apart. Keep your shoulders retracted (imagine popping your shoulder blades in your back pocket) and engage your lats (the muscles down the sides and mid back).

2. Take a deep breath in, brace your abs and make sure your knees are soft (not locked out). Start the movement by hinging at the hip, pushing your bum back as far as it can go and feeling the tension in the hamstrings (the muscles at the back of your thighs).

3. Maintaining a flat back and a neutral spine, keep your chin tucked in (imagine you are holding a tennis ball under your chin) and slowly lower the weight down to mid shin, keeping the knees soft throughout (we want to avoid locking the knees).

4. At the lowest position, start to exhale, squeeze your bum and drive the floor away with your heels to come up to full extension – in other words, hips fully straight, right back to where you started, standing up nice and tall.

Which muscles are you working?

Your posterior chain (everything running down your back)
Bum (glutes)
Legs (predominantly hamstrings and calves)
Back and shoulders (trapezoids, lats and erector spinae)
Core (abdominals and obliques)

Great for . . .

- Whole-body strengthening, because it works so many of the muscles we use in our everyday lives.
- Sedentary people, because it fires up those weak glutes.
- The strength transfers into other sports, giving you power and stability when running.
- Fat-burning, because it's complex and requires so many different muscles.

Training tip

Don't rush it, this one takes time to master. You want to get a good range of motion before you increase the intensity by adding more weight. You need to feel the tension primarily in your hamstrings not your quads.

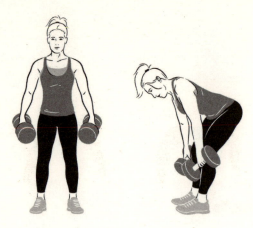

Romanian deadlift

Variations

This is different from a conventional deadlift because your legs stay slightly straighter. It could also be described as a stiff leg deadlift, and you will feel greater tension in the hamstrings, although you don't want to lock your knees – keep them soft. The aim here is to push your bum back as far you can, as if you were opening a door behind you with your glutes. Feel the hamstrings lengthening, keep a nice neutral spine with your chin tucked in and then squeeze the glutes to come up to full extension at the hip, standing up nice and tall.

Why do it? You will be hinging with a slightly greater range of motion because your legs are straight. It relies less on the quads than a conventional deadlift, and is great for hamstrings.

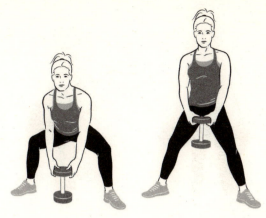

Sumo deadlift

This deadlift requires a wider stance, so stand with your feet spaced a bit further apart and with your toes pointed slightly outwards and near your groin. Still keeping your lats engaged with your shoulders back and down, bend at the hips to reach down and grab the weight with both hands. As you come down to grip your weight, your chest will be facing forward, due to your hips being a little lower because of the wider stance.

Why do it? It's a great workout for your hamstrings, and can be a good alternative to a conventional deadlift if you have difficulty with lower back pain.

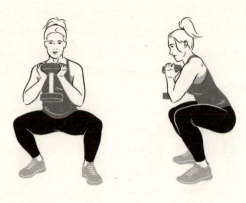

Squat

What is it?

The squat is another incredibly effective compound move that builds overall strength and stability. It's used by professionals as a performance marker for power, strength and mobility. It's also a hugely functional move we use in our everyday lives.

How to do it

1. Start with your feet about shoulder-width apart, heels firmly on the floor. If you are just using your body weight, your arms can stay by your sides. If you are using weights, hold them tight at each shoulder.

2. With your chest proud and shoulders back, take a big deep breath in, brace your core and start the movement by hinging at the hip, pushing your bum

back slightly as you begin to descend, driving your
knees out towards the corners of the room. It may
help your balance when doing a body weight squat to
hold your hands in prayer at your chest, or reach your
arms out in front of you, returning them to your sides as
you stand up.

3. Aim to keep the weight in your heels throughout the
movement. Ideally you want to get your bum lower
than your knees at the lowest point of the squat. Keep
driving the knees out, keep that abdominal brace and
don't let your knees go over your toes.

4. At the bottom of your squat (wherever your mobility
allows), squeeze the glutes, drive your heels through
the floor, keeping the chest proud and hips and chest
raised. Exhale as you drive up to full extension at the
hip, right back to where you started, looking straight
ahead.

Which muscles are you working?

Bum (glutes)
Legs (mainly quads, but also hamstrings)
Core (abdominals and obliques)

Great for . . .

- All-round lower body strength and power.
- Improving posture.
- Sedentary people as it works the glutes and hip
  flexors.
- Possibly improving hip mobility.

Training tip

You are aiming to get a full range of motion as you drive lower towards the ground. This can take some time to achieve. Really focus on mastering the move before you take on any weights or variations.

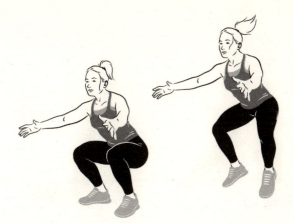

Plyometric squat

Variations

This is the dreaded jump squat and is quite advanced! You're turning up the intensity a notch by adding a jump out of the squat. This generates more power from that bottom position, but be careful with the landing; it needs to be soft to minimize impact, so if you are making a lot of noise, maybe this move isn't for you just yet. As you exhale to come out of the squat, you are springing into the air so that both feet leave the ground. Be careful if you have pre-existing knee problems – you want to try to land gently before moving into the next rep.

Why do it? It's a great cardio workout because plyometric squats are so taxing and leave you out of breath pretty quickly. The explosive movement will help to increase your strength, speed and power.

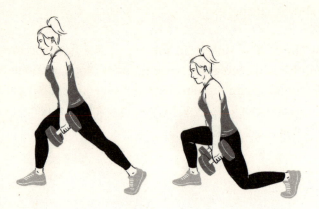

Bulgarian split squat

This is a great single-leg movement, with the back leg providing support and stabilization for the front leg, which is doing the work. Start from a standing position, bring one leg back so you're in a split stance or a lunge position, back foot positioned with your toes flexed to support your front leg, feet still just about shoulder-width apart. Then lower yourself into a deep lunge, dropping the back knee right down to just about kiss the floor. You want to keep a neutral spine, so you may feel like you are slightly leaning into that front knee but you want to ensure your front knee isn't tracking over your toes. Once you are at the bottom of this split stance squat, drive up using predominantly your front leg, and return to the split stance position, being careful not to lock out at the knee. You have the option to increase the intensity by elevating the back foot on a low, stable surface or even your sofa, but when doing so, make sure all of the above still applies.

Why do it? The Bulgarian split squat is a fantastic lower leg strengthening exercise because it doesn't load as much on the back. It's useful for building leg strength and single-leg stability. You can add in a weight when you master the move.

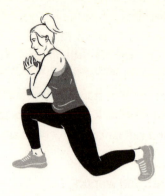

Reverse lunge

What is it?

The lunge is an exceptional exercise for developing lower body strength, up there with the squat. You can execute a lunge in a variety of planes: stepping one leg in front, behind or to the side. Personally, I prefer the reverse lunge because it tends to · place less pressure on the knees. If you have space, you could make the movement dynamic by doing walking lunges.

How to do it

1. Start with your feet about shoulder- to hip-width apart. Take a breath in and take a big step behind you, with that back foot confidently making solid contact with the floor and kissing the back knee down on the floor if your hip mobility allows.

2. Keep the spine neutral; you may feel like you are slightly leaning towards the front leg. Check that the front knee is tracking just over the mid-foot.

3. Brace the core, squeeze the glutes, exhale and push the floor away with that back foot to come up to full extension at the hip, standing up nice and tall and bringing the foot back to the start position. Take a big breath in and repeat on the other side.

Which muscles are you working?

Bum (glutes)
Legs (quads, hamstrings and calves)
Core (abdominals and obliques)

Great for . . .

- Lower body strength, because it works primarily on one leg at a time.
- Identifying whether you have one side / leg weaker than the other, which can help improve the bilateral movement (the squat).
- Core strength, because you use your core muscles to maintain stability and control during the move.
- Improving balance and posture.

Training tip

Make sure your knee doesn't travel forwards when you lunge; it should stay directly over the foot. You want to be moving your body straight downwards, not forwards.

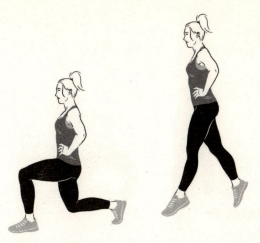

Plyometric lunge

Variations

You can turn up the intensity of this exercise by performing a plyometric variation, aka the jumping lunge. At the bottom of the lunge, push both feet off the floor and jump, scissoring your legs so you end up with the other foot behind. This is one to be cautious about if you have pre-existing knee problems.

Why do it? You get amazing cardiovascular benefits as plyometric lunges are so tiring, and you'll challenge your dynamic stability and coordination too. This is my least favourite exercise in the whole world, but I know it's good for me, especially to improve my running ability.

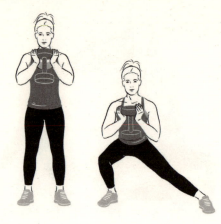

Lateral lunge

Also known as a side lunge, where you step out to the side before lungeing, rather than behind. Ensure you are maintaining a stable connection with the floor with the stepping foot, and focus on stabilizing the ankle to produce power on the working leg.

Why do it? It works the frontal plane of your body (side-to-side movements), which is often neglected in training programmes. The lateral lunge is easy to get wrong or to rush, thereby negating the benefits, so really focus on your form.

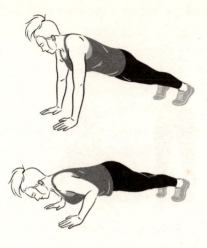

Press-up

What is it?

The press-up is one of the ultimate benchmarks of upper body strength, but you have to get your technique right, a) so you are working the correct muscles and b) to prevent shoulder injury. Progress through the variations of the movement slowly. Don't worry about mastering a full press-up on your toes straight away.

How to do it

1. Start in a plank position, making sure you position your hands just outside your torso, aligned with your chest. Your back should be flat and your spine neutral. Retract your shoulders and keep your core tight.

2. Take a breath in and start to lower your body to the floor, keeping your back flat and your elbows tight to your body, not flaring out to the side of the shoulders. Your elbows want to be pointing just behind you.
3. At the bottom of the press-up, exhale and squeeze the glutes and abs. Push through your hands, the whole body raising at the same rate (again, with neutral spine), until you come up to straight and full arm extension.

Which muscles are you working?

Back (lats, rhomboids and trapezoids)
Shoulders (deltoids)
Chest (pecs)
Arms (triceps)

Great for . . .

- A total upper body workout.
- Strengthening your shoulder joints.
- Beginners, as you can start on your knees before progressing to a full press-up (see variation on page 142).
- Tricep strength (think arm definition).

Training tip

The correct form is essential to make sure you don't take the hit in your shoulders. Think of it as very much a tricep-dominant exercise, where you are using the shoulders to stabilize. Start where you can move well and develop from there (see the variations on pages 142–143); don't feel the pressure to do a full press-up on your toes straight away as you may end up causing an injury.

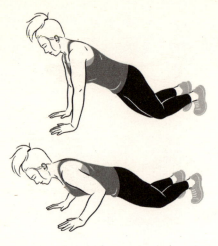

Press-up on knees

Variations

A beginner version, with knees down. Start on your hands and knees, walk your hands slightly forwards and lower your hips so that your back is flat and your spine is neutral; retract your shoulders and keep your core tight. Start to lower your body to the floor, making sure your hands are just outside of your body, aligned with your chest.

Why do it? Don't worry about needing to start here, as it is where I started too! It is pointless doing half-reps on your toes; far better to master this at full range first before progressing.

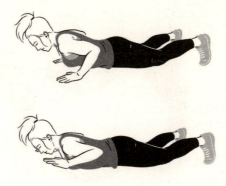

Hand release press-up

Start in a plank position as for a full press-up, then lower yourself right down on to your chest. Take your hands off the floor, then return them to the floor, exhale and push yourself up into the start position.

Why do it? I love this variation as it enables you to get really close to a full press-up, but it's slightly easier as it is done in two parts, giving you a few seconds of rest before you power back up.

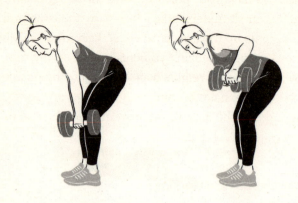

Bent over row

What is it?

The bent over row is a great move for working your upper body, by pulling a weight into your chest. Because you are standing in a hinge position, you are also working your core to support your body. It's essential to maintain strong form with this move.

How to do it

1. Holding a dumbbell in each hand, stand with feet shoulder-width apart.
2. Retract the shoulders and with soft knees, start to hinge at the hip (like the deadlift), pushing your bum back, loading the hamstrings, and with a flat back and tight core.

3. Once you have your position, with the weights directly under your shoulders, take a breath in and row (pull) the weights up towards your chest, keeping your elbows tucked in and squeezing your rhomboids at the top.
4. Slowly lower the weights back to the starting position with a slow exhale, keeping your muscles engaged. There should be little to no movement in the rest of the body during each rep.

Which muscles are you working?

Arms (biceps)
Upper and lower back and shoulders (trapezoids, lats and rhomboids)
Core (abdominals)

Great for . . .

- Building bicep strength.
- Strengthening your upper back and shoulders.
- Working on your lower back (because of your hinge position).

Training tip

Be careful not to round your back, especially when you get tired. Keep it straight.

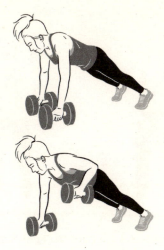

Renegade row

Variations

Start in a high plank position (arms extended), with your hands holding a pair of dumbbells, if possible. With a flat back, your shoulders over your hands and your feet as wide a base as you need, take a breath and, as you exhale, row (pull) one weight to your armpit. The challenge is to keep the hips solid without swinging from side to side. Lower the weight with control and switch sides.

Why do it? This is good if you find the bent over position hard on your lower back. You are also working your core to fight the rotation of the torso as you row each dumbbell.

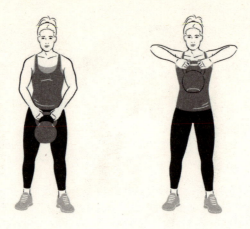

Kettlebell high pull

Hold the kettlebell with both hands against your body, arms extended, shoulders retracted. Take a breath, brace the core and, as you exhale, pull the weight up to just underneath your chin, ensuring your elbows flare out either side and finish above the weight. Then slowly lower.

Why do it?   This exercise is great for targeting muscles in your shoulders and back, including the trapezoids, mid-back rhomboids and deltoids.

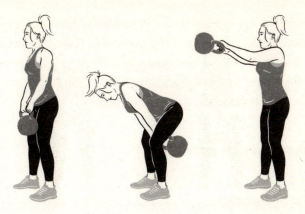

Russian kettlebell swing

What is it?

The kettlebell swing is a dynamic strength exercise that requires you to generate power through your posterior chain (the muscles at the back of your body), almost working your hips like a pendulum, propelling the kettlebell in front of your body, so it's weightless in your arms.

How to do it

1. Stand with feet hip-width apart, holding the kettlebell in both hands and with shoulders retracted.
2. Start the swing by pushing your bum back, with soft knees, and squeezing the glutes to push the kettlebell between your legs, then "snap" the knees back as you swing the kettlebell up to eye level, almost like a pendulum motion.
3. Ensure you keep a flat back and a neutral spine, with your chin tucked in throughout the movement.

4. Once you have enough momentum, the kettlebell should feel light in your arms; it's the glutes and hamstrings that are doing the work. However, do ensure that at the top of the swing you are not hyperextending the spine; squeeze the glutes hard at the top of the swing to maintain that neutral spine.

Which muscles are you working?

Bum (glutes)
Legs (hamstrings)
Shoulders and mid-back (lats)
Core (abdominals)

Great for . . .

- Building endurance.
- Working multiple muscle groups in one move.
- Improving posture.
- Burning fat because it's a dynamic move.
- Developing power in the glutes.
- Working both upper and lower body.

Training tip

Be cautious of swinging the kettlebell too high –
eye level is enough. You can minimize this risk by
focusing on squeezing your bum at the top of the
swing. You also need to be careful not to swing
back too much and hyperextend the back.

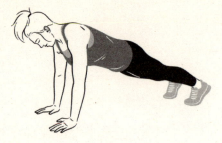

Plank

What is it?

The plank is the ultimate core challenge! You have to hold your body weight up so it challenges your core abdominals, obliques, shoulders, back, glutes . . . everything. It requires strength, endurance, and balance.

How to do it

1. Start on your hands and knees, then stretch your legs back one at a time so that you are supporting your body weight with your hands and toes. Make sure your shoulders are above your hands, and that your bum isn't in the air – we want to avoid any downward-looking dogs!
2. Ensure your back is flat, your shoulders retracted and your lats engaged.
3. Squeeze your bum and your abs and breathe deeply. Hold the position for as long as possible.

Which muscles are you working?

Core (abdominals and internal and external obliques)
Shoulders (deltoids)
Bum (glutes)
Legs (hamstrings)

Great for . . .

- Full body conditioning – there's hardly a muscle you don't use.
- Seeing progress: you can time yourself to see how long you can hold strong form.
- Low-impact strengthening.

Training tip

A really common mistake is to hold your bum high in the air. Keep your body as straight as you can.

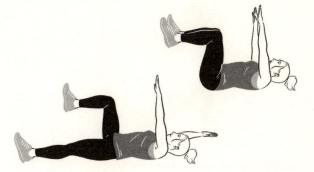

Dead bug

Variation

The dead bug is a fantastic exercise to work on your core control. It focuses on strengthening the muscles that stabilize your hips and spine. Lie on your back with your arms and legs above you, knees bent at 90 degrees, like in a table top position. Connect your back to the floor and then lower one alternating arm and leg at a time, working your core muscles. As you go through the reps of this movement, keep thinking about pushing your lower back into the ground. If you find that you are arching your lower back, reduce the range of extension of the arms and legs, or just take a rest and go back to it later.

Why do it? It's a real challenge to your anterior core and exceptional for stability – you use it to strengthen your lower back, thereby preventing excessive lumbar hyperextension (the big arch in your back).

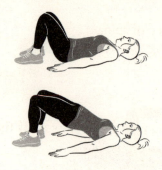

Glute bridge

What is it?

The glute bridge is an awesome body-weight movement that focuses on the hip extension movement. It is low impact, can be done anywhere and specifically isolates the gluteal muscles in your bum, the ones that get weak when we sit for too long.

How to do it

1. Lie down on your back and dig your heels into the floor just in front of your bum.
2. Lay your hands softly either side of your body.
3. Take a breath in and, as you exhale, drive your hips up into the air, squeezing the glutes at the top before slowly lowering the hips back down to the floor.
4. Keep your spine neutral throughout.

Which muscles are you working?

Bum (glutes)
Lower back (erector spinae)
Legs (hamstrings)

Great for . . .

- Strengthening your glutes, especially the largest one, the gluteus maximus.
- Giving your bum better definition.
- Working the hip hinge while lying on your back.
- Helping you to keep an upright posture.

Training tip

If you feel your hamstrings working too hard, move your feet nearer to your bum and think about keeping your core tight and squeezing your glutes a little tighter too.

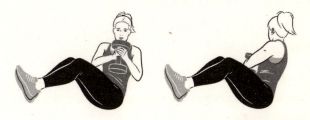

Russian twist

What is it?

The Russian twist is a fantastic exercise for the core, and is one of the few core exercises that uses rotation, unlike the basic crunch.

How to do it

1. Sit with your feet in front of you, knees raised and leaning back as far as you feel comfortable while keeping the spine neutral.
2. Rotate your arms all the way over to one side, then the other side.
3. Ensure your gaze follows the movement of the torso to maintain a neutral spine.

Which muscles are you working?

- Abdominals
- External and internal obliques

Great for . . .

- Working the core and obliques.
- Canoeists and rowers because it targets those key muscles you're using.
- Supporting your posture by working the core.

Training tip

Focus on range and control rather than speed. When you master the movement you can hold a weight in both hands or try raising your feet off the ground, knees together – or both!

LIFTING LESSONS

As with everything in life, you will come across a lot of people preaching or sharing different things they are obsessed with, or explaining that the latest fitness fad 'worked for me'. Well, good for them. It's important to follow the path that makes YOU feel good, that thing YOU love doing. Do more of that. For me it was about more than just lifting weights; this was a life discovery, working out who I was, what I wanted, what I stood for, and what I was willing to work hard at to achieve. They say you should try anything once, but I don't think I have ever known someone to try lifting and not become hooked on the feeling. It's about empowerment, believing and trusting in your body, investing time in ensuring it is as robust and healthy as possible for the daily routine.

I followed the crowd for years, while secretly enjoying my own weird and wonderful hobbies and, over time, I let society dictate who I was and what I wanted to be. It wasn't until I started to celebrate myself physically that I had the confidence to stand (relatively) tall and know exactly what my value and contribution was to this world. And it wasn't until I was faced with adversity, when my mum became unwell, that I realized just how important it was to follow my life's purpose, because if I didn't now, when would I? I allowed comparison to others rule my headspace. Life is too short to worry about a thigh gap.

Trust me, I know that the 'getting started' part of anything is really hard. So many 'what ifs', so much fear of failure, of doing it wrong, of someone judging you. But I always try to remember this: those who matter don't mind, and those who mind, don't matter. If we apply this to fitness, we start to remember who we are doing it for and focus on giving ourselves the best possible opportunity to succeed in life. Success for me isn't what jeans I fit into, it's the meaning of my actions and my relationships. Once I started to regularly work on myself, for myself, things changed. Something switched in me; I found I was capable of more. I didn't have to be like anyone else. I wanted to be like me.

My goals changed from things like 'lose 10 pounds' or 'fit into size 8 clothes' to 'develop glute strength', thus enabling me to squat better, which made me a better runner. 'Learn to do a handstand by Christmas' dispelled my fear of kicking upside down and gave me amazing shoulder stability and upper body push strength. When people ask me how much I weigh, or if I weigh myself, I can now genuinely say I don't know or care. What a revelation. I spent years of my life chasing my 'ideal' weight. And when I got there? I felt the same, maybe just a little tired – and hungry.

Everyone starts as a beginner, and being a beginner can be very daunting – if you don't have experience of something or you don't know what to expect you may find yourself coming up with reasons why you can't or shouldn't do it. So if I have managed to inspire you, start by grabbing your laptop or phone and googling some fitness classes or personal trainers in your local area. Alternatively, phone a friend and organize a long walk or run around the park or maybe a gym session together. The decision to get active will most likely be the best one you ever made.

This last year has truly been the making of me; after years of doubting my physical value, hard work and a successful career change mean that I now stand content, comfortable, happy, proud and excited about where I am at. So much so that I want to spend my life showing others that it really is possible to change your mindset, to physically turn your life in a new direction, surrounded by positivity and acceptance. But it has to come from you, you have to want it, you have to believe it's possible.

Here are some of my key learnings over the past year or so.

• If You Want Something, Ask For It

After years of being 'not good enough' (in my head), I've now learned that I make the decisions and I'm in control. If I don't like something, I can change it – I don't have to follow a crowd. So, ask for it. Ask someone out. Go to a new gym class. Call an old friend. Change career. Move house. Go to a run club. What's the worst that could happen?

• Speak And Act Kindly To Yourself

I've learned to take a compliment this year. Finding self-acceptance and physical contentment is so powerful, it radiates, and the energy you give out, you will get back. So try telling yourself how amazing you are.

• You Can't Be Available All The Time

I'm an 'always on' kind of person, and can respond, adapt, provide an answer/solution to most things pretty quickly, but to what end? It's human nature to want to help others (and that is so important) but make sure you are helping yourself too.

• Appreciate Effort, Not Results

If you are working hard and making a positive change, it is very natural to want to see or feel the results. If the effort level is consistent, you will be the result of what you put in, not that one time you ate a chocolate biscuit.

• Extreme Isn't Always The One

I've spent a lot of time going 'hard' after something, and celebrating when I get it quickly, but not everything in life needs to be a race. Now I take a more considered approach to my life – you really don't have to do it all.

• Cheer For Yo Damn Self!

We spend a lot of time observing the progress of others and waste a lot of headspace on things completely unrelated or useful to our own development. So appreciate the work you have put in, love your own personal journey, and don't compare.

• Don't Worry About It

I'm going to focus more on living in the moment, and not over-analyzing the potential outcome. Work with what you can control; as for the rest . . .

So, now it's all in your control; you decide, you have the power to commit to change or not. Anything worth having demands hard work, and the best project you could ever invest in, is your mental and physical health. No one else can do it for you, you have to lift yourself.

'IT REALLY IS POSSIBLE TO CHANGE YOUR MINDSET, TO PHYSICALLY TURN YOUR LIFE IN A NEW DIRECTION, SURROUNDED BY POSITIVITY AND ACCEPTANCE.'

References

1 Effect of exercise type during intentional weight loss on body composition in older adults with obesity; Beavers KM et al, *Obesity (Silver Spring)*, November 2017.

https://www.ncbi.nlm.nih.gov/pubmed/29086504

2 Resistance training and intra-abdominal adipose tissue in older men and women; Hunter GR et al, *Medicine & Science in Sports & Exercise*, June 2002.

https://www.ncbi.nlm.nih.gov/pubmed/12048332

3 High-intensity resistance and impact training improves bone mineral density and physical function in postmenopausal women with osteopenia and osteoporosis: The LIFTMOR randomized controlled trial; Watson SL et al, *Journal of Bone and Mineral Research*, February 2018.

https://www.ncbi.nlm.nih.gov/pubmed/28975661

4 Exercise dosing to retain resistance training adaptations in young and older adults; Bickel CS, Cross JM, Bamman MM, *Medicine & Science in Sports & Exercise*, July 2011.

https://www.ncbi.nlm.nih.gov/pubmed/21131862

5 Treatments for mild to moderate depression; NICE, April 2018.

https://www.nice.org.uk/guidance/cg90/ifp/chapter/treatments-for-mild-to-moderate-depression

6 Association of efficacy of resistance exercise training with depressive symptoms: meta-analysis and meta-regression analysis of randomized clinical trials; Gordon BR et al, *JAMA Psychiatry*, June 2018

https://www.ncbi.nlm.nih.gov/pubmed/29800984

7 A comparison of the effects of hatha yoga and resistance exercise on mental health and wellbeing in sedentary adults: a pilot study; Taspinar B, Asian UB, Agbuga B, Taspinar F, *Complementary Therapies in Medicine*, June 2014.

https://www.ncbi.nlm.nih.gov/pubmed/24906581

8 The effects of a session of resistance training on sleep patterns in the elderly; Viana VA et al, *European Journal of Applied Physiology*, July 2012.

https://www.ncbi.nlm.nih.gov/pubmed/22045416

9 Changes in arterial distensibility and flow mediated dilation following acute resistance vs. aerobic exercise; Collier SR et al, *Journal of Strength & Conditioning Research*, October 2010.

https://www.ncbi.nlm.nih.gov/pubmed/20885204

10 Twice-weekly progressive resistance training decreases abdominal fat and improves insulin sensitivity in older men with type 2 diabetes; Ibañez J et al, *Diabetes Care*, March 2005.

https://www.ncbi.nlm.nih.gov/pubmed/15735205

11 Mediation of cognitive function improvements by strength gains after resistance training in older adults with mild cognitive impairment: outcomes of the Study of Mental and Resistance Training; Mavros Y et al, *Journal of the American Geriatrics Society*, March 2017.

https://www.ncbi.nlm.nih.gov/pubmed/28304092

12 Does strength-promoting exercise confer unique health benefits? A pooled analysis of data on 11 population cohorts with all-cause, cancer and cardiovascular mortality endpoints; Stamatakis E et al, *American Journal of Epidemiology*, May 2018.

    https://www.ncbi.nlm.nih.gov/pubmed/29099919

13 The impact of sleep deprivation on food desire in the human brain; Greer SM, Goldstein AN, Walker MP, *Nature Communications*, February 2014.

    https://www.ncbi.nlm.nih.gov/pmc/articles/PMC3763921/

Further reading and useful websites

You are officially invited to join TEAM LIFTED UK! I have created a private Facebook group, for people like you: an online community of people from all over the UK and beyond, brought together by our love of wanting to be the best we can be. We have a true mix of experiences and abilities; we discuss training tips, nutrition and lifestyle hacks, and just generally celebrate conquering life together. Making a decision to pursue a healthier and fitter lifestyle can feel quite lonely sometimes, so we will always be on hand to give you that little push you may need to get it done! Just search TEAM LIFTED on Facebook, request to join and I will be there ready to bring you into the fold. Introduce yourself to everyone and give a little hello and you are off! I can't wait to meet you.

Women's Health UK, a fantastic magazine and digital publication, has some excellent hints and tips for training, sample workouts and nutritional support. They have various blog posts and training plans, some of which I have been fortunate enough to contribute to. Check out their Instagram page @womenshealthuk.

Maybe a podcast could be your thing? One of my idols is strength coach Joslyn Thompson Rule. She has a podcast called *Fitness Unfiltered*, and I have spent many hours listening and nodding my head to her discussions and debates with some very inspirational people. Find her on @joslynthompsonrule or search *Fitness Unfiltered* in your podcast app.

Some other Instagram inspo for home and gym workouts:

@bradleysimmonds
@london_fitness_guy
@twicethehealth
@aliceliveing
@britishwl

Getting serious about weightlifting? You may want to search for a local powerlifting or weightlifting gym. British Weight Lifting is the governing body for lifting in the UK and has information on how to get started in lifting, including finding your nearest club, plus information on campaigns and competitions. www.britishweightlifting.org

If pure weightlifting isn't for you but you feel you would like the intensity and the competitive element of team training, perhaps CrossFit might be an option. I have found that Cross-Fit boxes all have a slightly different vibe, as it is totally driven by the owners, the coaches and the members. Don't be afraid to start – the good boxes will welcome you. The good thing about CrossFit is that all workouts should be scalable to any ability. Search for your local box on their website. www.crossfit.com

If you fancy giving modified strongman training a go, like me, here are my top picks for places to go and train in London:
The Foundry London @foundryfit and www.foundryfit.com
The Commando Temple @commandotemple and www. bestronger.co.uk

Charities and governing bodies
The NHS provides guidelines on health and fitness.
www.nhs.uk

Sport England is an organization that aims to inspire people into sport. Twice a year it produces the Active Lives survey, which measures adults' activity levels. They are the team behind THIS GIRL CAN, the national campaign to break down the barriers to exercise, aiming to show all women that fitness can be for them. @officialsportengland and www.sportengland.org

Women in Sport is a UK charity that aims to get more women into sport through its research and campaigns. @womeninsport_uk and www.womeninsport.org

And finally . . . you can get in touch with me
You can find me on Instagram at @laurabiceps. Here I share an insight into my training world and personal life, with some useful videos and workout inspiration. You can also meet my LIFTED community on Instagram by using the hashtag #team-lifteduk or at @lifted.ldn. You can also find my home of fitness at Ministry of Sound @ministryofsoundfitness, where we have a full timetable of sessions if you are in and around London.

If you are outside London, or if group fitness isn't your thing, there is a huge range of commercial gyms all over the country, all with different vibes and styles. Why not experiment until you find one that suits you?

If going to the gym really isn't your thing, then make your living room, your garden, the local park or just the great outdoors your gym. Exercise and fitness really should be accessible to all in whatever way you choose to do it. Join a local yoga class or dance fitness class, or put on a Davina McCall DVD (this is where I first started all those years ago!).

You could also check out the hashtags #womenwholift and #strongwoman on Instagram for some pretty extreme inspiration! It is incredible to see the passion and energy for this kind of training, but remember never to compare: this is YOUR journey, they are on theirs, and they are not you, so find your own path and cheerlead along the way.

Acknowledgements

This book is dedicated to my two best friends: my mum aka 'Mummy Biceps' and my dad 'DJ-Hog'. The smartest, most caring, selfless, loving and supportive parents in the world. No matter what I told them I wanted to do in life, they always told me to 'just go for it, darling' and they would cheerlead me the whole way. My number one fans, thank you for everything you have sacrificed for me, I love you both so much.

Thank you to the other half of our small but mighty family unit: Wendy, Martin, James and Sophie. Granny and Grandpop Smith are watching us in admiration from afar! Your support means the world to me.

To Julia, Emily, Rachel and the whole team at Penguin Life: thank you for seeing something in my coaching that could be shared with the world, to potentially help to shape the decisions people make day to day, to feel confident with who we are, and to work to ensure that we are the best we can be, building the foundations for a wonderful fit and healthy life!

To Alice, Francesca, Daisy and Nora at Found Entertainment: thank you for taking me under your wing to help grow and develop my passion, and to share experiences, learnings and professional teaching to others.

To PJ and Neil, who gifted me their gym to start LIFTED on a Sunday afternoon at CrossFit Hammersmith. 'I wish someone had helped me when I first started personal training. When you are up and flying, pass it on to someone else.' (PJ Cavalli, owner.)

To the legends Ben Gotts, Dave, AliMck, Will and Anna-Maria, and everyone at The Foundry, you really are 'Where the Strong Belong'. You have taught me to be not only physically strong, but mentally strong too. Deflecting all your terrible banter is a constant challenge.

To Olivia and Harry at Ministry: thank you for taking a chance on me from the beginning. I so desperately knew LIFTED could be a 'thing' so to be able to coach and inspire everyone in the Ministry of Sound Fitness studio is an absolute honour.

To Shane Collins, for teaching me to feel confident being a purple cow. Because no one notices a brown cow, but a purple one, you're going to stop and take a photo and send it to a friend.

To all my friends, who over the years have put up with me spending more time at the barbell than at the bar, and listened to my exhausting chat about gains, WODS and AMRAPS. Sarah and Kate: I know you know about getting a perfect shot of my nourishing coffee for 'the gram' – I thank you! Katie and Nat, for your athletic running partnerships. Jenan for your fantastic work on the prowler.

To my ex who taught me to never settle. Cheers for your friendship and the life lessons.

And to every single one of you who have perhaps unknowingly inspired me in the gym, with your visible ambition, lifting for the first time, working outside of your comfort zone, moving with purpose and tenacity, cheering on others working alongside you. You may be the reason that someone else starts or doesn't quit. Keep paying it forward.

Laura, aka 'Biceps'
xoxo